PREVENTION'S BEST™
America's #1 Choice for Healthy Living

HEALING HERBS

Natural Medicine at Its Best

By the Editors of *Prevention* Health Books

RODALE

ST. MARTIN'S
PAPERBACKS

W9-BVF-709

The information in this book is excerpted from *Herbs That Heal* (Rodale, 1999).

Prevention's Best is a trademark and *Prevention* Health Books is a registered trademark of Rodale Inc.

HEALING HERBS

© 2000 by Rodale Inc.

Cover designer: Anne Twomey
Book designer: Keith Biery

ISBN 0–312–97584–8 paperback

Printed in the United States of America

Rodale/St. Martin's Paperbacks edition published November 2000

St. Martin's Paperbacks are published by St. Martin's Press, 175 Fifth Avenue, New York, NY 10010.

10   9   8   7   6   5   4   3   2

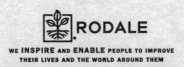

RODALE

WE INSPIRE AND ENABLE PEOPLE TO IMPROVE
THEIR LIVES AND THE WORLD AROUND THEM

Notice

This book is intended as a reference volume only, not as a medical manual. The information given here is designed to help you make informed decisions about your health. It is not intended as a substitute for any treatment that may have been prescribed by your doctor. If you suspect that you have a medical problem, we urge you to seek competent medical help.

Jean L. Fourcroy, M.D., Ph.D.
Past president of the American Medical Women's Association (AMWA) and past president of the National Council of Women's Health in New York City

Clarita E. Herrera, M.D.
Clinical instructor in primary care at the New York Medical College in Valhalla and associate attending physician at Lenox Hill Hospital in New York City

JoAnn E. Manson, M.D., Dr.P.H.
Associate professor of medicine at Harvard Medical School and codirector of women's health at Brigham and Women's Hospital in Boston

Mary Lake Polan, M.D., Ph.D.
Professor and chairperson of the department of gynecology and obstetrics at Stanford University School of Medicine

Elizabeth Lee Vliet, M.D.
Founder and medical director of HER Place: Health Enhancement and Renewal for Women and clinical associate professor in the department of family and community medicine at the University of Arizona College of Medicine in Tucson

Lila Amdurska Wallis, M.D., M.A.C.P.
Clinical professor of medicine at Weill Medical College of Cornell University in New York City, past president of the American Medical Women's Association (AMWA), founding president of the National Council on Women's Health, director of continuing medical education programs for physicians, and master and laureate of the American College of Physicians

Carla Wolper, R.D.
Nutritionist and clinical coordinator at the Obesity Research Center at St. Luke's–Roosevelt Hospital Center and nutritionist at the Center for Women's Health at Columbia-Presbyterian Eastside, both in New York City

Contents

Introduction

There has been a revolution in self-healing.

It began in backyard gardens, porch planters, windowsill boxes. It mixed the magical with the practical, poetry with medicine. Its lifeblood was lore handed down through the generations. And its heart was growth and soil.

You've heard plenty about it: the herbal revolution. But what you may not have heard is that it offers lots of satisfactions beyond healing. Herbs can also relax you, stimulate you, and add taste, scent, color, and texture to your life.

This book is your tour guide to that world. You'll learn how to use herbs medicinally for dozens of common conditions, among them dock root for anemia, guggul for high cholesterol, and nettle for muscle cramps. You'll even discover which herbs can help you quit smoking.

You'll also find out how to use basil to pass a test, mugwort to have pleasant dreams, and an apple to look younger. You'll relax with herbal massage oils as well as learn which herbs to use for symptoms ranging from anxiety and arthritis to ulcers and varicose veins.

This book gives you practical ideas for maintaining

your health, youth, and joy in living, in addition to hundreds of specific uses for herbs.

Every new journey has its cautions, of course, and so does this one: When using herbs medicinally, never combine them with prescription drugs unless you check with your doctor first. Likewise, herbs alone can't treat serious or chronic illnesses. And don't use herbs if you're pregnant or nursing unless a medical doctor gives you the okay. In general, use them in combination with a healthy lifestyle, professional medical care, and the counsel of an herbal expert when you need it.

Remember also that herbs, like all medicinal remedies, can have side effects, so please read the precautions in the Safe Use Guidelines for Herbs and for Essential Oils section at the back of this book before treating yourself.

Now let's get to the fun part: Good reading and good health!

PART ONE

The New Age
of Herbs

Herbs as Modern-Day Healers

Suddenly, herbs are everywhere you look. In health food stores, drugstores, and even supermarkets, echinacea sits next to cold and flu decongestants. Plants with names so magical they sound perfect for casting spells, such as ginkgo and black cohosh, line the shelves. You'd think we were witnessing a breakthrough in modern medicine. But these "modern" remedies have healed people for thousands and thousands of years.

Herbs were used to cure ills ranging from aches and pains and menstrual problems to insomnia and depression centuries before modern medicine invented drugs. Here are just a few of the ways in which herbs have helped to heal people throughout the ages.

- Garlic, which doctors acknowledge has cholesterol-reducing powers, dates back at least 5,000 years as a healing gem.
- People in ancient Africa applied the gel from the aloe plant to wounds from poisoned arrows, and people of India utilized it as a cooling agent.

- Herbalists 2,000 years ago recommended using ginseng to enlighten the mind and brighten the eyes. Current herbalists prescribe the herb as a tonic that enhances mental function.
- Native Americans took echinacea to treat snakebites, fevers, and stubborn wounds. Early American settlers adopted the plant as a home remedy for colds and flu.
- Soldiers in the Trojan wars treated their wounds with yarrow—a plant used today for cuts and scrapes.
- The women of ancient Greece drank wine in which chasteberry leaves had been steeped to regulate their menstrual cycles.

Since the dawn of time, our ancestors depended on plants to nourish them and keep them well. Then, about a hundred years ago, people decided it was time for a change. We turned our backs on our ancient relationship with herbs and looked elsewhere for our food and medicine.

Now, like prodigal children, we're returning to herbs—in huge numbers. More than 30 percent of the U.S. population relies on herbal alternatives to medically approved drugs. In just a 2-year period, sales of echinacea jumped 72 percent, while sales of the depression fighter St. John's wort skyrocketed 1,900 percent.

We have a plethora of herbs to choose from, as well as items the herbal healers of yesteryear could never have imagined: St. John's wort lipstick, essential oil chewing gum, herb-laden energy bars. Companies now sponsor major ad campaigns to promote the sale of herbs. Behind this revival are millions of people who are looking to herbs as a natural source of healing and comfort.

A Natural Connection

Often through trial and error, the early herbalists began to understand Mother Nature's products and their healing powers. Using intuition, experience, and common sense, they made good use of the plants that the earth gave them. "If someone has a burn, you are going to look around and choose a plant that is succulent and juicy—like aloe," says Ginger Webb, the herbal education coordinator for the American Botanical Council in Austin, Texas.

These wise herbalists passed on their knowledge to others, who then added their own experiences to it, eventually creating what we know—and sometimes disregard—as folklore. Folklore ensures that important information filters down to future generations by weaving instructions into a good story—something easy to remember and interesting enough to tell over and over again.

The craft of healing with herbs flourished until the late 19th century. The Industrial Revolution and new technology then gave birth to the idea that anything nature can do, man can do better. Where the earth gave us meadowsweet and willow bark as pain relievers, science gave us a much stronger medicine in aspirin.

Then came the discovery of penicillin, which led some to believe that a "magic bullet," a manmade miracle medicine, could cure all our ills, says Ellen Evert Hopman, a professional member of the American Herbalists Guild (AHG) from Amherst, Massachusetts, and author of *Tree Medicine, Tree Magic* and *A Druid's Herbal for the Sacred Earth*. People started to turn away from herbs.

Naturally, after a few generations passed, a good deal of herbal history was lost. And after nearly a half-century of our overusing penicillin and other antibiotics, bacteria are developing immunities to these drugs. Many diseases and infections are becoming harder to cure, notes Hopman.

How to Make a "Green" First-Aid Kit

Daily life is peppered with minor medical annoyances like cuts, scrapes, and digestive distresses. Fortunately, herbs help treat them and provide you with fast, effective relief. A variety of medicinal plants act as wound healers, infection fighters, and antiseptics.

Here is what you'll need to put together your very own herbal remedies kit, as recommended by Claudia Cooke, M.D., a holistic doctor in New York City.

- Aloe. Apply the gel from inside the plant to minor burns, sunburn, and rashes. At home, keep a plant on a sunny windowsill. For travel, carry a tube of aloe gel.
- Arnica. To ease the pain, swelling, and discoloration of bruises, spread on arnica gel. Don't use on broken skin.
- Dried calendula flowers. An effective wash for cuts and scrapes. Make a freshly brewed strong tea with 1 tablespoon of petals per cup of boiling water. Steep for 20 minutes, strain, and cool. Then use it to wash the cut.

Coming Full Circle

Today, many people find themselves returning to the herbal ways of their ancestors, says Feather Jones, a professional member of AHG and director of the Rocky Mountain School of Botanical Studies in Boulder, Colorado.

Why are we seeking solace in herbs again? The reasons are as numerous as the herbs themselves, but here are a few of the major ones.

A feeling of empowerment. Many of us have been educated to believe we must hand over our health to another

- Dried chamomile flowers. Chamomile tea eases digestive discomfort, calms anxiety, and relieves mild insomnia. For eye infections such as pinkeye, strain the flowers from a freshly brewed tea through a coffee filter and allow the tea to cool. Then use it as a wash.
- Echinacea tincture. Good for treating colds, flu, and infections. For infections, dilute the echinacea in an equal amount of water and apply to the affected area.
- Gingerroot or capsules. For nausea or motion sickness, take ginger as a tea or in capsules or chew it in its crystallized form.
- Goldenseal powder in capsules. Open a capsule and sprinkle the contents onto an infected cut.
- Tea tree essential oil. Dilute the tea tree oil with vegetable oil to fight fungal and bacterial infections in cuts, abrasions, and athlete's foot.
- Witch hazel tincture. Protects broken skin from infection. Cleans wounds and aids healing of rashes and minor burns.

person—specifically a doctor. But herbalism allows us to take charge of our own well-being. We can use herbs to stay healthy and prevent sickness. We can even use plant medicines to treat illnesses. "It is very empowering to realize that you can depend on yourself and take care of yourself and your family with herbs," Hopman says.

Further, herbal medicine sometimes has advantages over conventional: In some cases, you can treat what mainstream science cannot. "Conventional medicine falls short when it comes to treating chronic conditions and everyday illnesses like cold and flu. People with those problems are increasingly taking care of themselves with herbs," notes Hopman.

Getting back to nature. In a high-tech world where computers are far more common than gardens, some people feel cut off from their life source. They don't spend as much time with plants, flowers, and wildlife as they would like. Using herbs reconnects them with nature. "It returns a part of yourself back to the earth," Jones says.

Herbalism gives us a new sense of intimacy with the plant world around us. "The more you learn about herbalism, the more amazing it becomes. You learn that a flower growing along the side of the road is a medicinal plant. And that the weeds growing in between your spinach and your tomatoes are medicinal plants. It raises your consciousness," Webb says.

Herbalism connects us with our environment in another way. Because both we and plants are part of the natural world, our bodies instinctively know what to do with herbs. "You are giving your body something that is a known entity. We have evolved with plants, so our bodies know how to read an herb as opposed to a pharmaceutical," Webb says.

A need for gentle and affordable care. When scientists started creating more potent, synthetic versions of herbs in the early part of the 20th century, people didn't foresee side effects and the fallout from their use, Jones says. Afraid of the overpowering action of pharmaceuticals, many people want the milder, yet just as effective, option of herbs.

On a practical level, herbs sometimes offer refuge from the expensive and tangled world of conventional health care. Trips to doctors, specialists, and pharmacies all add up financially. In some cases, herbs help offset those costs. "People are tired of side effects; they are tired of the expense of going to the doctor and getting a prescription," Jones notes.

Whatever the reason, self-care with herbal medicine is a powerful experience. For some, it evolves into a way of life, not just a way of healing. "If you start taking tinctures and teas, your lifestyle changes. You don't just take a pill. You help make your medicine. For instance, herbal teas have this wonderful aroma. You slow down to boil the water and steep the plant. You start experiencing your medicine in a different way. You are part of it," Webb says.

Picking and Choosing Made Easy

There's no need to feel overwhelmed and confused by a store shelf stocked with a dozen brands of echinacea. Strange-sounding herbs, such as dong quai or skullcap, need not daunt you. As an experienced shopper, you already have extraordinary skills. Bring them along when you're choosing your herbal products, whether in a health food store, a discount drugstore, a mail-order catalog, a supermarket, a local gym, or the Internet.

When you buy groceries, you don't usually select items off the shelf on impulse. First you make a shopping list by determining what you need. By the same token, you shouldn't randomly select a handful of medicinal herbs without knowing what their benefits are and how well they match your needs. Herbs can play a vital role in improving and maintaining your health if you choose and plan wisely. Do some research before you shop. Then make a list. Here are some guidelines from herbal practitioners to help you.

Understand the power of plants. Since antiquity, medicinal herbs have been used to relieve throbbing headaches and heal minor cuts, scrapes, and burns. They can provide a surge of stamina or kick your digestive system into gear. Certain herbs assist your immune system in reducing fevers and fighting parasites. Some brighten your mood; others spice up your sex life. Still others help you with emotional stress.

Many prescription and over-the-counter products contain medicinal ingredients that are derived from, or similar to, those found in plants. For instance, acetylsalicylic acid, better known as aspirin, is similar to salicin, a pain reliever found in willow bark. Progesterone-like substances for birth control pills were derived from compounds found in Mexican yams.

Respect the medicinal powers of herbs. "Definitely treat herbs as you do medicine," says Mindy Green, a founding and professional member of the American Herbalists Guild, director of educational services for the Herb Research Foundation in Boulder, Colorado, and coauthor of *Aromatherapy: A Complete Guide to the Healing Art.*

Although most herbs are safe, with few or no side effects, herbal experts caution that some can be toxic if taken in the wrong form or in large quantities. Especially when you're using an herb for the first time, it's wise to begin with the lowest recommended dosage. And watch for side effects before you consider increasing the amount, cautions Angela Stengler, N.D., a naturopathic physician and herbal author in Oceanside, California.

Comfrey, for example, is excellent when used externally as a poultice for sprains and bruises, but it can cause cancer or liver damage if taken orally.

Choose the herb that's right for you. Before you buy an herb, make sure it's suitable for the condition you're treating.

"When someone wants to use herbs for the first time, I recommend trying one herb for a specific need instead of buying a half-dozen," says Dr. Stengler. "See how your body interacts with this herb. Is it giving you the desired

Supplements or Fresh Herbs?

Many herbs offer culinary delight when sipped in teas, sprinkled on foods, tossed in salads, or cooked in stews, but in most instances, the amounts are far too small to give you any real medicinal benefits, says Angela Stengler, N.D., a naturopathic physician and herbal author in Oceanside, California. That's where supplements come in.

For instance, a crushed clove of garlic added to pasta sauce delivers satisfying aroma and taste, but studies show you would need up to five cloves of garlic per day to lower your blood pressure and cholesterol. You can gain the same therapeutic benefits more conveniently by swallowing standardized extract garlic capsules or tinctures.

If you're looking to improve your memory and circulation, ginkgo is an ideal herb choice. But, again, supplements provide more medicinal value than a cup of tea made with fresh or dried ginkgo.

Most studies indicate that you need to take 60 to 240 milligrams (24 percent standardized extract) of ginkgo to achieve the medicinal benefits needed to sharpen your memory and enhance circulation. To match that amount, you'd need to drink up to 15 cups of ginkgo tea a day.

Eating herbs for flavor is fine. But for treating specific health conditions, herbs eaten in foods cannot match the therapeutic values of supplements.

effect? Are there any side effects? Get to know the herb. What it looks like. How it works."

Know the versatility of herbs. Certain herbs provide both culinary delight and medicinal benefits. Fresh cloves of garlic enliven a dish of clams and linguine, but garlic may also help prevent major cardiovascular disease when used in appropriate amounts over specified periods of time. Sage is another culinary spice that, when used medicinally, works effectively as a gargle for sore throats.

Know the limitations of herbs. Herbs work effectively for the occasional headache or sleep-interrupted night, colds, the flu, or the rash you got from hiking in woods laced with poison ivy. Botanical medicine can even contribute to optimal health when it's used correctly as part of an overall wellness program, says Dr. Stengler. But botanicals alone cannot be expected to solve all health problems, especially major ones such as heart disease, high blood pressure, diabetes, or cancer.

Don't expect miracles. Herbs, like vitamins and prescriptions, won't make up for lack of exercise or poor eating habits. Herbs work best when you incorporate nutritious foods and regular exercise into your lifestyle.

Learning the Herbal Lingo

It could be a shopper's nightmare: aisles and aisles of herbs. Some in tiny glass bottles. Others in capsules. Some fresh, some dried. Still others are in teas, chewing gum, throat lozenges, salves, and ear drops.

On the other hand, if you know where to begin, it could be a shopper's paradise.

Let's begin right here, by learning the benefits and drawbacks of selecting herbs in five basic forms: tinctures, teas, capsules, powders, and poultices.

Take a tincture. Tinctures are extracts made by steeping herbs in alcohol. They work best when you need quick absorption. "They are especially helpful for people who have trouble absorbing nutrients because of digestive problems," explains Dr. Stengler. "Tasting the herb stimulates digestion and body processes."

Depending on the herb, you can use a tincture internally or externally. Most tinctures are made with diluted alcohol (100 proof) or a mixture of 50 percent ethanol and 50 percent water. Nonalcoholic tinctures made with glycerin are also available. Either type can be taken directly by mouth or added to water, juice, or herbal tea for better palatability. When stored in a cool, dark place, a tincture can last for several years without losing strength. Tinctures don't always taste great, however, and they aren't routinely standardized.

Sip some tea. A popular way to take medicinal herbs is by drinking a small amount of fresh or dried herb in a steaming cup of tea. Most herbal teas contain high concentrations of volatile oils, but they take time to make and may not be as potent as tinctures or capsules.

Still, herbal teas have one huge advantage: They usually taste great. For your favorite herbal blends, consider buying herbs in bulk that have been organically grown and are free of commercial fertilizers. These herbs should smell fresh, be free of mold, and nearly match the color of fresh herbs. Store them in airtight containers away from sunlight.

Swallow a capsule. Herbs in capsule form are often standardized and offer convenience. If you have difficulty swallowing pills, the capsules can be opened and the contents stirred into food or liquids. It takes the body longer to absorb a capsule than a tincture, however. And if there is no expiration date on the label, it can be difficult to judge freshness.

Sprinkle on powder. You can easily add herbs in powder form to food or beverages to provide a direct effect on your throat and gastrointestinal system. For example, adding a teaspoon of slippery elm to your morning oatmeal will

Get More Power from Your Tea

How you brew a cup of herbal tea affects its medicinal strength. As opposed to simply steeping a tea bag for a few minutes, *infusions* and *decoctions* maximize herbs' healing powers.

You make an infusion by steeping 1 ounce of fresh or dried herb leaves and flowers in 1 pint of boiling water for 10 to 15 minutes. Herbalists regard infusions as simple rituals that unite a healer (you) and a healing substance (the herb) with a healing intention ("I want to get a good night's sleep," for instance).

A decoction is similarly created by simmering 1 ounce of tough herb parts (usually the roots, bark, dried berries, or seeds) in 1 pint of boiling water, usually for about 10 to 20 minutes. This long simmering process coaxes out the plant's medicinal properties.

To make a decoction to curb a cough, for instance, place 1 teaspoon of fresh or dried licorice root, crushed or chopped, in a glass or stainless steel pot with a lid. Add 1 cup of water. Bring to a full boil, then reduce the heat to the lowest setting and let the root simmer gently for about 20 minutes. Keep the pot covered. Strain the decoction through a fine-mesh plastic strainer into a glass jar. Press the herbs in the strainer with the back of a wooden spoon to extract more of their liquid. Licorice is an anti-inflammatory, antiviral herb that soothes coughs. You can drink up to three cups per day.

help soothe a sore throat or relieve heartburn, according to Dr. Stengler. The downside of powders is that they are hard to standardize unless the powder comes from a capsule.

Apply a poultice. A poultice is a layer of crushed herb, fresh or dried, that is dampened and applied directly to the affected area of the body. Normally, a layer of cotton, such as cheesecloth, is placed between the herb and the skin. A poultice provides relief to external parts of the body only. For instance, if you burned your forearm, a calendula poultice would speed the healing of your skin. You would not use a poultice, however, to relieve a cold, says Dr. Stengler.

Decoding the Label

Package labels are supposed to make our lives easier. The labels on herbal products don't. By law, they cannot carry medicinal claims or post possible side effects unless these have been proven in tests that cost millions of dollars and require years to undertake.

Since plants can't be patented, it doesn't make financial sense for companies to spend millions of dollars establishing evidence that ginger, for instance, helps in digestive complaints. The Food and Drug Administration classifies herbal products that have not been through its drug premarket approval process as dietary supplements, not drugs.

Even with vague labeling, however, consumers can navigate effectively through the herbal product aisle with the following tips.

Learn both the botanical and common names of the herb. Knowing the botanical, or Latin, name gives you an extra edge when making a purchase. It guarantees that you're buying the right type of herb for your needs. Depending on where you live, an herb answers to several names. The hormone-balancing herb that eases menstrual discomfort is known as chasteberry as well as vitex. And some herbs, such as echinacea, come in several types. The savvy shopper seeking relief from a cold would know to ask for *Echinacea purpurea* and not *Echinacea angustifolia*, according to Dr. Stengler, because the former has been the subject of more research.

Buy brands that are standardized. This assures that you get the same dose of the active ingredient every time. It says so on the label. The potency of herbs can vary from batch to batch, plant to plant, place to place, and time to time. Buying standardized avoids guesswork. But be aware that most herbs aren't available in standardized form, so you may need to rely upon other factors, such as those listed below, to help make your selection.

Look for expiration dates and safety seals. To ensure full potency of capsules, buy only products that post an expiration date. Without a date, you cannot be sure how old the capsules are. Also, buy products with safety seals for added protection.

Seek the recommended dosage. Manufacturers' recommended dosages vary from one product to another, so it's a good practice to check the label before taking the herb. Note if the instructions tell you to take the herb with meals or in between meals.

Choose organic. The label should clearly state if the product was made free of chemical fertilizers. Most certified organic products are processed according to standards outlined in the California Organic Food Act of 1990. Some products include that information on their labels as well.

Check the ingredients. The label should display the amount of every active ingredient. Make sure that the product does not contain any ingredient you may be allergic to. Also, check for any fillers or preservatives that may have been added.

Choose single-herb products. You may like that multivitamin you take every day, but when it comes to selecting herbs, experts recommend that you avoid buying multi-herb products. By taking several herbs blended into one product, such as a capsule, you may get inadequate doses of each.

Buy proven herb brands. Select herbs from brands that have been tested. These brands are backed by solid research. Examples include Kwai garlic, Ginkgold ginkgo, Thisilyn milk thistle, and Kira St. John's wort.

Look for cautions. Many reputable manufacturers list special precautions, such as the best time to take the product (with meals or in between) and when you should avoid it (if you are pregnant or have a specified medical condition, for example).

More Is Not Better

When it comes to herbal remedies, less is often best. You may think you need a dozen different herbs a day, but you could probably get the same results with only a few herbs—and at much less cost, says Amy Rothenberg, N.D., a naturopathic physician in Enfield, Connecticut.

In fact, certain herbs can cancel out the effectiveness of others. Some herbs—including immune system boosters like echinacea—can lose their effectiveness when taken every day for too long a time. Others, such as kava kava, can cause side effects when used for weeks on end. And when you're taking a whole slew of herbs, you don't know which ones are actually making you feel better and which ones are not helping at all.

Steer clear of miracle claims. Avoid buying herbal products that claim they contain "secret formulas" or "miracle cures." If an herb sounds too good to be true—and lacks scientific backing—it probably is.

Find the manufacturer. By law, the manufacturer's address must be included on the label. Manufacturers who provide telephone numbers and Web site addresses build their credibility with consumers.

Using Herbs Safely and Wisely

Proper use of medicinal herbs is essential. To ensure a safe and effective experience, herbal experts offer these tips.

Use herbs only when needed. Home herbal remedies should be used only when necessary and only in appro-

A better strategy is to limit yourself to just a few herbs that can treat more than one problem at a time. Mullein, for example, can help yeast and urinary tract infections, digestive complaints, and skin problems.

Consider also that the best remedies for some health problems do not come from herb gardens. If you get infections, for instance, it could be because you're eating too much sugar, which can suppress your immune system. Or maybe you're not eating enough vitamin- or mineral-rich foods. Problems like insomnia, tension, and lack of energy could be improved with exercise, yoga, or relaxation techniques such as meditation or deep breathing.

The bottom line: A combination of just a few herbs and other natural therapies can often be the key to relief.

priate amounts. This is not an area where a "more is better" philosophy applies. For example, echinacea works most effectively when taken at the onset of a cold to lessen its severity. But taking echinacea every day all year long may lessen its potency.

Rely on knowledgeable experts. Learn about herbs, and talk them over with either your doctor or some other qualified health care practitioner who has training and experience in using herbs medicinally. That might be an M.D. or D.O. (medical doctor or doctor of osteopathy) trained in herbal medicine or an N.D. (naturopathic physician) trained in botanical medicine. Or it might simply be an herbalist who knows the historical and current uses of herbs, understands how herbs work in our bodies, and often prepares herbal products for clients. Just be sure the herbalist is open to coordinating your care with your physician.

Several organizations can provide you with names of qualified herbal practitioners in your area. These organizations include the American Herbalists Guild, P.O. Box 70, Roosevelt, UT 84066; the American Association of Naturopathic Physicians, 601 Valley Street, Suite 105, Seattle, WA 98109-4229; the National Commission for Certification for Acupuncture and Oriental Medicine, 11 Canal Center Plaza, Suite 300, Alexandria, VA 22314; and the American Holistic Medical Association, 6728 Old McLean Village Drive, McLean, VA 22101.

Know when to stop. Pay close attention to instructions on how long to take an herb. Some suggest you take a break for several weeks or months before resuming. Others can safely be taken every day. Sometimes the recommended time depends upon the condition. You should expect some improvement in an acute condition, such as a cold or the flu, within 24 to 48 hours, says Dr. Stengler.

If the condition is chronic, such as arthritis or

menopausal hot flashes, you may need to observe your symptoms for up to 2 months to feel any difference, Dr. Stengler says. If your health condition does not improve after using the herbal remedy for a reasonable amount of time, seek medical help. Certainly, see your doctor if your condition worsens.

Keep your doctor informed. According to the *Journal of the American Medical Association*, 15 million Americans take herbs and prescription medicine at the same time. But 60 percent fail to tell their doctors that they are taking herbal remedies. Inform your doctor so he can be on the lookout for possible drug–herb interactions.

Store herbs properly. Place dried herbs in airtight glass containers and store them in a cool, dark place. They will retain their potency for up to 6 months this way. For tinctures, dark glass bottles guarantee potency for several years. As for capsules, check for an expiration date and store them in a closed jar away from heat and sunlight.

Feel-Good Therapies

The fundamental uses of herbs are healing, cooking, and having fun.

That's right. *Having fun*. It's not all serious business. Herbs can heal you, but they can also bring you lots of enjoyment. Think about how they stir the senses—smell, touch, taste, sight. Imagine the lingering aroma of a lavender essential oil candle; the silky, rich sensation of a rose-infused massage oil; the sugary taste of angelica candy; the bright, beautiful colors of a floral potpourri.

Still, they're actually medicines, aren't they? Well, that depends on your point of view. Herbs have a healing effect, but when was the last time a bottle of aspirin brought the words "pampering" and "self-indulgence" to mind?

It's true that, for some people, modern herbalism has simply become a substitute for traditional medicine. Think of all they're missing. They treat their bodies, but what about their minds and their spirits? Herbs can enrich people's daily lives in so many more ways, says herbalist Rosemary Gladstar, director of the Sage Mountain Herbal

Education Center in East Barre, Vermont, and author of *Herbal Healing for Women.*

Open yourself to a new world and experiment with all the different facets of herbology. Treat yourself to an herbal foot massage, cook up some herbal candies, cool down with a relaxing herbal-scented spritzer. In other words, have fun!

Aromatherapy

Through the senses of touch and smell, aromatherapy may help to erase the physical, emotional, and spiritual roadblocks we face every day. Aromatherapy uses essential oils, which are extremely concentrated aromatic oils distilled from plants. "It literally takes hundreds of pounds of plant material to produce a small amount of essential oil," Gladstar says.

People who practice aromatherapy say that each essential oil has specific healing properties. For instance, the scent of peppermint oil alleviates indigestion and nausea, rosemary treats lung congestion and sore throats, and sandalwood counters inflammation and hemorrhoids. Avoid rosemary if you have hypertension or epilepsy.

According to aromatherapists, this aromatic art works in two ways. First, it operates through inhalation. We've all experienced scents that influence our moods and emotions. Aromatherapy goes one step further. The theory is that specific scents trigger more than just feelings; they also incite internal chemical reactions that can enhance your immune system or reduce tension, says Mindy Green, a founding and professional member of the American Herbalists Guild (AHG), director of educational services for the Herb Research Foundation in Boulder, Colorado, and coauthor of *Aromatherapy: A Complete Guide to the Healing Art.*

Second, essential oils work topically, entering your body through your skin. To use oils in this way, pour them into baths, add them to massage oils, or apply them with compresses. "It isn't just the odor. There can be 500 different compounds in one oil. It has therapeutic properties that affect our entire systems," Gladstar says.

Many people turn to aromatherapy because of its simplicity. To get started, purchase 100 percent natural essential oils. Start your collection, Gladstar says, with three basic oils that have wide ranges of application: peppermint, chamomile, and lavender. Peppermint treats stomach problems, headaches, congestion, and muscle spasms, and it can be used as a natural stimulant. Chamomile may reduce indigestion, premenstrual syndrome, muscle inflammation, stress, and insomnia. Lavender is a wonderful emotional healer; it helps treat nervousness, exhaustion, insomnia, irritability, and even depression.

People with sensitive skin can have allergic reactions to essential oils, even when they're used externally. To be sure you're not one of them, first do a patch test. Put 10 to 12 drops of essential oil in an ounce of massage oil or unscented body lotion. Dab a bit of this mix on an inconspicuous place, such as your inner arm or the back of your neck at the hairline. Over the next 12 hours, check for redness or itching. If either occurs, use a weaker solution or try another oil.

Because they're so concentrated, essential oils can be toxic if you ingest them, so don't take them internally. It's also easy to overdo them with even a small amount, so always dilute any oil before applying it to the skin. Dilute essential oils with carrier oils, which are neutral, nonaromatic oils such as almond, jojoba, or grapeseed oil.

Here are some suggested recipes for using essential oils:

For massage/body oils, 10 to 12 drops (from a standard medicine dropper) per ounce of carrier oil; for baths, 3 to 15 drops per bathtub; for inhalants, 3 to 5 drops per bowl of hot water; for room sprays, 20 drops per 4 ounces of water; for compresses, 5 drops per cup of water.

Waiting to Inhale

When using aromatherapy, you need to decide how you want to disperse the aroma into the air or onto your body. Here are popular options.

Diffusers heat essential oils and spread their scent into the air. A basic ceramic diffuser has a saucer at the top into which you drop oil and water. Directly underneath the saucer is a votive candle. The candle warms the oil and water, emitting essential oil vapors into the room. A more complex electronic diffuser uses an air pump and an atomizer. For aromatherapy in your car, buy a diffuser that plugs into your cigarette lighter. You'll create a relaxing refuge during a traffic jam or a rough commute.

Lamp ring diffusers are small ceramic rings that fit around a lightbulb. You place essential oils and water inside the ring. Heat generated by the bulb warms and diffuses the oils.

Mists are essential oil mixtures in spray bottles. You can buy them or make your own by mixing oils, vodka, and distilled water. They can be sprayed in the air to scent a room or sprayed on your body.

Aromatherapy candles come in many different sizes and types. You can buy candles scented with just one oil or a mixture specially created to promote a specific mood, such as relaxation, sensuality, or meditation.

Baths and Hydrotherapy

People have been tapping into the healing powers of water for at least 6,000 years. Cold baths energize and stimulate. Room-temperature bathwater has been called nature's finest tranquilizer. The classic hot bath eases muscle spasms and relaxes the body and mind. Even ice and steam can comfort a variety of everyday ailments.

Nothing can make you feel better than a long, hot bath can—nothing but a long, hot bath accentuated with herbs and essential oils, that is. "Baths are one of my favorite things. Therapeutically, it is like immersing your body in a giant cup of tea," Gladstar says. From the water, your skin absorbs the healing and soothing properties of herbs. They enhance the water's ability to relax you, soothe sore muscles, rejuvenate dried skin, and ease congestion from a cold.

To make an herbal bath, start with a strong tea. Place two or three handfuls of an herb or herbal mixture into 2 to 3 quarts of boiling water. Cover it tightly; let it cool to room temperature and then strain it. Pour the herbal tea into a full tub of water, says Green.

Which herbs are good for baths? Just about any one, as long as it has a pleasant aroma, Green says. Avoid using large amounts of "hot" herbs like clove, cinnamon, ginger, or cayenne, she cautions. They can irritate the skin. She recommends that beginners start by experimenting with calming and sweet-smelling herbs, such as lemon balm, chamomile, rose, or lavender.

To use essential oils in a bath, Green suggests starting with geranium, orange, or lavender. You can use 3 drops of orange and up to 10 drops of geranium and lavender. For an ailment such as a cold, use 5 to 8 drops of eucalyptus oil. To get the full effect of an herbal bath, Green suggests soaking for at least 20 minutes.

Orange oil is phototoxic—if you use it, even diluted, in

areas of skin that are exposed to the sun, it can cause uneven pigmentation. So reserve it for times when you won't be going out immediately into the sun. Don't use eucalyptus oil for more than 2 weeks; it's best added to 1 teaspoon of vegetable oil, then added to the bath.

If you don't have time to linger in a bath, you can still enjoy the soothing effects of herbs and water by making an herbal salt scrub to use in the shower, Gladstar says. Buy some natural sea salt at a health food store and pour it into a wide-mouth glass jar. Leave about 2 inches of space at the top. Pour almond oil over the sea salt until the jar is nearly full, then add two to five drops of essential oil, preferably lavender or lemon balm. When you're taking your shower, grab a handful of the salt and vigorously rub your body with it. Be gentle if you have sensitive skin. Then proceed with your regular shower. "This is done in expensive spas. You wash off all the dead cells in your skin, and you stimulate your circulation. Your skin is glowing and soft. It is marvelous," Gladstar says.

Cough Medicines

Although it takes a bit of cooking time, there's something to be said for making your own cough medicine. Herbal cough syrups are herbal decoctions and infusions—basically teas made by a long, slow simmering process. They not only soothe harsh coughs but also give you that special sense of satisfaction that always seems to come when you create something from scratch. "You always make better medicine at home. You have much more control over quality, how strong it is, the flavors. You have your own good intentions in that medicine," Gladstar says.

Take 1 teaspoon every hour or so, advises herbalist Betzy Bancroft, a member of the AHG and manager at

Herbalist and Alchemist in Washington, New Jersey. You can make syrups from fennel, coltsfoot, licorice, mullein, marshmallow, or wild cherry bark.

To make the syrup, combine equal parts of any of these herbs in tincture form (except use only one-half part wild cherry bark); add an amount of honey equal to the combined tinctures. If you want more flavor, add one-half part fruit concentrate, which you can buy at a health food

Cooling, Herbal-Scented Waters

How would you like to have your own portable oasis? There's nothing like spraying your body with cool, herbal-scented water to take the edge off an exhausting day or hot, muggy weather.

Sprays made with peppermint, lemon balm, and cucumber oil are naturally cool and refreshing, says herbalist Rosemary Gladstar, director of the Sage Mountain Herbal Education Center in East Barre, Vermont. You can easily make your own to keep in your purse or briefcase, car, and office.

Purchase a 4-ounce dark bottle with a twist-off spray pump at a beauty supply store. Using a small funnel, pour 1 tablespoon of vodka into the bottle (the alcohol acts as a preservative). Pour distilled water into the bottle until it almost reaches the top. With a dropper, add three to five drops of essential oils. To enhance the cooling effect, use peppermint, lemon balm, orange, or cucumber essential oils. Shake the bottle before each use. The mixture should keep indefinitely. Don't use it on broken skin or spray it in your eyes.

Note that peppermint oil and lemon balm may cause skin irritation or an allergic reaction in people with very sensitive skin.

store. Store the mixture out of the refrigerator. Shake it well before using.

Gladstar offers this recipe: First, make an herb tea. For a cough medicine to calm a hard, dry cough, mix one-half part valerian, one part mullein, one part licorice root, and one part wild cherry bark. Crush or chop the herbs. Place 4 ounces of the mixture per quart of water in a glass or stainless steel pot. Bring the liquid to a rolling boil and then reduce the heat to the lowest setting and let the decoction simmer for 10 to 20 minutes. Keep the pot covered so that the herbs' essential oils don't escape. Steep overnight in the refrigerator.

To make the syrup, simmer the decoction until it's reduced to a pint (2 cups) for every quart of water you used. This will give you a concentrated, thick tea. Strain out the herbs. Pour the liquid back into the pot. For each pint, add 1 cup of honey. Warm the honey and liquid together until they mix well. If you desire, add 3 to 4 tablespoons of brandy per half-pint. Brandy acts as a preservative and relaxes throat muscles. Refrigerated, the syrup should last a few weeks.

Flower Essences

It sounds like a commercial, but it's true: If you want to express your feelings to someone, whether of love, grief, regret, or joy, there's almost no better way to do it than with flowers. The connection between flowers and emotions seems eternal, and people who use flower essences take this idea deeper. They believe that certain flowers possess a special ability to heal emotional hurts. Whereas essential oils capture the physical healing power of plants, flower essences capture their emotional healing power. Consider flower essences the "soul" of plants, Gladstar says.

To make a flower essence, place a perfect flower in a glass or crystal bowl filled with spring water. Then set the bowl on the ground near the mother plant. After a few hours in the sun, remove the flower with a small twig and add the water to a small bottle filled halfway with brandy.

The first flower essences created were the Bach Flower Remedies, discovered by British immunologist, bacteriologist, and pathologist Edward Bach, M.D. Dr. Bach believed that emotional distress is the underlying cause of physical illness. He also believed that flowers have the ability to treat emotional problems and, therefore, prevent or cure diseases.

Each of his 38 Bach flower essences is supposed to treat a specific emotional condition. For instance, the flower essence cerato helps people who have trouble making decisions and who constantly seek advice from others. Gentian aids those who get discouraged easily or who become filled with self-doubt after every small setback. Water violet is for people who like to be alone and who are independent, talented, capable, clever, calm, and self-reliant. It's interesting that many of the flowers Dr. Bach used are actually blossoming herbs.

You'll find flower essences in health food stores. Just trickle a few drops on your tongue or add a few drops to a small glass and slowly sip. You can also add some flower essence into your bathwater or pour a few drops into a spritzer bottle filled with water. Gladstar always takes a spray bottle of Rescue Remedy—Dr. Bach's famous five-flower combination for relieving stress—with her when she flies. "I do it to keep centered and focused and happy," she says.

Candies and Lozenges

If flowers don't catch your interest, then how about candy? Herbal candies can be good for you, and they taste good, too. Some contain blends such as peppermint, thyme, sage elder, and horehound, while others combine lemon with mint, essential oils, and even vitamin C. The old standby sore throat and cough drop contains the herb eucalyptus. Gladstar remembers when, as a child, she enjoyed Jump for Joy balls and horehound candies and lozenges made from powdered herbs.

You can find many of these candies at drugstores and health food stores, but you can also make your own. Here's how: For candy, choose herbs that have a pleasant taste or scent, perhaps angelica and fennel. Lozenges are just medicated candy. One combination that is effective against sore throats uses sage, fenugreek, licorice, or slippery elm, Bancroft says.

To make candy or lozenges, place 1 cup of a decoction or infusion designed for the illness you want to treat in a glass, ceramic, or stainless steel pan and add ½ cup honey or sugar. Simmer over low heat, stirring occasionally with a spatula or wooden spoon. Continue cooking the syrup until it is thick enough to coat the back of the spoon. Test it by dropping a small amount onto wax paper. As it cools, it should harden and hold its form.

Use ½ to 1 teaspoon of syrup for each candy or lozenge. After the candy has cooled and hardened, wrap each piece in plastic wrap, then store it all in a cool place. The pieces will keep for several months.

Massage Oils

It is instinctive for us to touch ourselves or another person when we're in physical or emotional need. Without thinking, you rub your temples if you have a headache, knead your calves if they're cramped, and put your arm around someone's shoulder if she's troubled. That's why therapeutic massage works so well. It's an expression of a basic human impulse. "Massage itself is therapeutic. Everyone needs more touching—foot massage, hand massage, a back rub," Gladstar says.

By adding herbs to massage oils, you can intensify this nondrug approach to relieving tension, reducing stress, and easing muscle pain. Certain herbs also help with skin care.

To make your massage oil, first choose a carrier oil. Good carrier oils for massage include almond, apricot, and grapeseed. Then decide which essential oil you want to use. For a relaxing massage, Gladstar recommends rose, lavender, chamomile, and comfrey. You can use them singly or mixed together.

For muscle pain and strains, Green suggests rosemary, juniper, and wintergreen. To loosen tight, cramped muscles, try sage. For dry skin, make a calendula massage oil.

After choosing your herb or herbs, place 2 ounces of dried herbs in a wide-mouth jar. Pour a pint of carrier oil over the mixture so that at least 2 inches of oil sits above the herbs, Gladstar says. Let it stand in a warm place and shake it every day for 2 weeks. Using a kitchen strainer or cheesecloth, strain the oil. Store it in your refrigerator and warm it in a pan on the stove before using.

The oil should last for several months, but don't keep it for more than a year. If you like, you can also add a few drops of an essential oil to the mixture. Use about 10 to 12 drops of essential oil to each pint of carrier oil.

If you need the oil quickly, place the herbs and oil in a double boiler, Gladstar says. Cover it with a tight-fitting lid and bring it to a slow simmer. Slowly heat the mixture for 45 minutes. Check frequently to make sure the oil doesn't get too hot. If it starts bubbling or smoking, reduce the heat. Strain the oil and then add a drop or two of an essential oil to enhance the aroma.

Skin Care

In 1400 B.C., an Egyptian queen was buried with tiny pots that are believed to have held her precious cosmetic creams and oils. During the second century, the ancient Roman doctor Galen created a recipe for face cream, possibly the first ever recorded. Made up of oils, wax, and water, it is a formula some herbalists still use today.

It makes perfect sense to use natural products to promote your own natural beauty. "Your skin is your largest organ of elimination and assimilation. Using herbs nourishes the skin and helps develop a radiance," Gladstar says.

Natural ingredients are useful in almost every aspect of your skin-care regimen. Cleansing soaps, facial steams, shampoos, astringents, creams, and beauty masks all originate from herbs and plants. Many commercial skin-care and cosmetic products contain herbs, but that doesn't make them true herbal formulas.

"A lot of herbs are being used in products that are not natural by any means. You need to be discriminating," Gladstar says. Look for products containing natural ingredients that you recognize. Too many chemical names in the ingredient list is a tip-off that the product is not natural.

If you have skin that has lost its luster, herbalists recommend two time-honored techniques: cleansing scrubs and toners.

Some herbal scrubs are gentle enough to use every day on your face and body. They clean, soften, exfoliate, draw out dirt, and smell great.

Herbalists say that it's important to apply a toner after scrubbing. Versatile and fragrant, toners promote circulation, soften, and help restore the skin's natural acid mantle. This slightly acidic surface, which is often washed away by harsh soaps, plays a crucial part in protecting your skin from bacterial invasions.

To restore vibrancy to your skin, incorporate this two-step herbal strategy into your daily beauty regimen with an easy-to-make scrub and toner.

You'll need the following equipment: a food processor,

Making a Henna Paste

If you don't want to go gray but are leery of regular dyes, henna might be just the thing for you. Henna powders of all shades are readily available at health food stores and through mail-order catalogs.

Here are the facts about henna, according to herbalist Rosemary Gladstar, director of the Sage Mountain Herbal Education Center in East Barre, Vermont.

- No matter what color you choose, all hennas contain some red. So if you're blond, expect red highlights.
- Unless your hair is super dirty, it's best not to shampoo before applying the henna.
- After application, henna will seem to be a full shade brighter than you expect. But it will fade dramatically after the first washing.
- Henna shades last about 2 to 3 months.

Now, here's how to apply henna.

- Select the right amount of henna for your hair length—2 to 3 ounces for short hair and 4 to 6 ounces for shoulder-length or longer hair.
- Mix the henna with boiling water to make a thick paste. Aim for a consistency similar to cooked oatmeal, not too dry and not too runny. Let the paste cool before applying.
- Dampen hair thoroughly and towel-dry.

clean coffee grinder, or blender; a large mixing bowl; a wire whisk; and a quart jar with a tight-fitting lid. You'll also need the following ingredients: 1 cup of ground oatmeal from rolled oats, ¼ cup of ground almonds or poppy

- Before applying henna, put on plastic gloves to avoid stains on your hands.
- Massage a small amount of olive or jojoba oil into your hair.
- Cover your hair completely with the henna paste. Your hair should feel like a thick helmet on your head.
- Cover your hair with a shower cap, plastic wrap, or plastic bag. Then hold it in place with a turban-wrapped towel.
- Depending on your shade of hair, leave the henna in for 30 minutes to 2 hours. The darker your hair shade, the longer you leave the henna on.
- Wash your hair with your normal shampoo and de-tangling rinse.
- Pick an old towel or T-shirt to dry your hair because the henna will leave stains.
- Let your hair air-dry before you brush.
- Remember, you won't see any shade differences until your hair is completely dry.

Note: If you have light-colored hair (blond, light brown, silver), always choose a lighter shade of henna, such as neutral to strawberry blond. Leave the henna in your hair for approximately 30 minutes. You might want to test it on a few strands before applying it to your entire head.

seeds, 2 cups of cosmetic clay, and 2 tablespoons of ground dried lavender, roses, calendula, comfrey, or chamomile (or any combination of these herbs).

To make your scrub, first grind the oatmeal to a fine powder in the food processor, coffee grinder, or blender. Place the powder in the mixing bowl. Then grind the almonds or poppy seeds to a fine powder and add to the bowl. Next, add the clay and herbs to the combined ground oatmeal and nuts or seeds. Mix thoroughly with the wire whisk. Pour the mixture into the jar and put on the lid. (The mixture can be stored for up to a year.)

To use your scrub, pour out 2 tablespoons of the mixture into your hands, add water to make a thin paste, and scrub your face and upper body gently. The selected ingredients soothe your skin, lift away dirt, exfoliate, and even clean your pores. Rinse and follow with a toner.

To make your toner, you'll need the following equipment: a pint-size glass jar with a tight-fitting lid, a fine-mesh strainer, a large mixing bowl, a measuring cup and spoons, a funnel, and eight plastic bottles with tight-fitting lids. You'll also need apple-cider vinegar, witch hazel, distilled water, and your choice of one or several herbs from the following list: comfrey leaves, plantain, calendula, red roses, chamomile, nettles, lemon balm, lavender, scented geranium leaves, mullein, yarrow, rosemary, and thyme.

Start by packing your chosen herbs into the jar. (If you're using dried herbs, fill the jar halfway; if you're using fresh herbs, loosely layer them to the top of the jar.) Next, pour in the vinegar and close the lid tightly. Let the liquid steep for 3 to 6 weeks, then pour it through a strainer into a bowl. Add 2 tablespoons of witch hazel to the strained vinegar. Pour ¼ cup of this mixture into each plastic bottle, and top each bottle with 2 cups of distilled water. Shake well before using.

The mixture will last for up to a year. Remember to refrigerate the bottles you aren't currently using. Don't worry if a slimy coating appears on the surface. Just remove it—it doesn't affect the quality of the toner. Apply the toner with a cotton ball or pad. You can also store the mixture in a misting bottle and spritz your face and body whenever you need a pick-me-up.

Preparing an herbal facial steam is one of the easiest ways to treat your skin, and it does wonders. Bring 2 to 3 quarts of water to a boil in a large pot. Toss in a healthy handful of an herb or herbal mixture.

For dry-to-normal skin, Gladstar recommends chamomile, roses, comfrey, lavender, and calendula. For normal-to-oily skin, she suggests sage, comfrey, calendula, and rosemary. Cover the pot, and let the water simmer for a few minutes. After you remove the pot from the heat source, place it on a stable surface, cover your head with a large towel, and put your face about 12 inches over the steaming brew, being careful not to spill the hot water. Steam for 5 to 8 minutes. When you're done, rinse your face with cold water and follow with a good moisturizing cream. Try this facial steam once a week.

Hair Rejuvenators

Centuries before you could buy hair coloring in a box, people were washing away gray—naturally.

Natural dyes work like commercial shampoo-in color treatments, but they get their hue-changing power from compounds in plants, not from chemical coloring agents. As with all hair coloring, it's important to select an herbal gray hider carefully, based on your original hair color and how much gray you want to cover.

For dark hair that's just beginning to sprout streaks of silver, a rinse with a strong cup of sage or rosemary tea can restore your original, deep shade, says Shatoiya de la Tour, an herbalist and founder of Dry Creek Herb Farm and Learning Center in Auburn, California. To make the tea, put 2 teaspoons of either herb in a cup of just-boiled water. Steep until cool, strain out the herbs, and use the liquid as a rinse after shampooing. Don't rinse this colored rinse out. Your hair should darken after several applications.

For hair that's brown, auburn, or medium to dark gray (not all white), try this strong herbal tea rinse. To 8 cups of boiling water, add ¼ cup each of dried nettles, sage, and rosemary; ½ cup of black walnut hulls; and two black tea bags, suggests beauty expert Stephanie Tourles, a licensed aesthetician in Hyannis, Massachusetts, and author of *The Herbal Body Book*. Steep for 3 hours and strain. Then add 2 teaspoons of sweet almond or olive oil and chill the mix in the refrigerator. Wash and rinse your hair, then put on rubber gloves and apply ½ cup of this mixture. Let it sit for a minute. Don't rinse; just towel-dry your hair with a dark towel that won't show stains. Use this treatment daily for 2 weeks, then as desired, recommends Tourles.

You can enhance your natural hair color by artfully applying henna, an herbal hair coloring made from powdered privet leaves (for blond and red hair) or from powdered indigo (for black hair). Henna hair-coloring kits come in a wide variety of subtle shades. Choose a hue that accentuates your natural hair color.

Potpourri

In some circles, potpourri is referred to as recreational aromatherapy. Potpourri is a simple art, used more to make a room smell nice than to treat medical conditions. "Having a pleasant fragrance around you is really uplifting, especially since we are bombarded with so many nasty smells," Bancroft says.

Potpourri has become increasingly popular, with sprays and flower mixtures available at department stores. But some contain artificial ingredients and synthetic oils, which can be harsh on your skin and your senses. Since potpourri is easy to make, you may as well use the natural and safe scents Mother Nature gave us, Green says.

The simplest way to create potpourri is to make a sachet. Pick flowers from your garden or herbs that you like, dry and crush them, and place them in a small cloth bag. If you don't have a bag, sew two pieces of cloth together and stuff it with the dried herbal mixtures, Bancroft says. Another easy potpourri technique is to simmer various herbs and plants in a pot of water on the stove. The scent will fill the air in moments. Popular plants used in potpourri include angelica, bay leaves, lemon balm, lavender, marjoram, and rosemary, although you can use whatever scents and herbs you enjoy.

PART TWO

Herbal Know-How

50 Herbs You Should Know

How would you like to make friends with a plant? Or, better yet, with 50 of them? Herbs won't feed your cat while you're off cruising the Caribbean, of course, but they will always be there for you when you need them most. They can protect, strengthen, relax, or invigorate you. They can spice up your meals, and they can lace the air around you with delicate scents. They're great to know.

Making new friends and developing relationships takes time, of course. And that's half the pleasure. When you first meet a new botanical, study it. Use it. Familiarize yourself with its shape, aroma, and healing powers. Feel how it interacts with your body before trying another, says Angela Stengler, N.D., a naturopathic physician and herbal author in Oceanside, California.

Each of the herbs you're about to meet has an enduring safety record, demonstrated effectiveness (often backed by scientific studies), preventive qualities, and popularity among the top herbal practitioners.

These herbs can help in all the areas of your life. Some of them help rev up your body's immune engine against invading viruses. Others assist in cleansing key organs, such as the liver. Some help restore hormonal balance. For women, cramp bark can ease menstrual cramps, while black cohosh can cool menopausal hot flashes. For your emotional needs, St. John's wort can chase away mild depression. Peppermint can aid in digestion by reducing flatulence and abdominal cramps. For your beauty and pampering needs, it's hard to resist a relaxing lavender bath or a skin-cleansing herbal facial.

"Herbs nourish our entire being, not just the physical body. They nourish our cells with their nutrients, and they nourish our inner being with their strength and beauty," says herbalist Rosemary Gladstar, director of the Sage Mountain Herbal Education Center in East Barre, Vermont, and author of *Herbal Healing for Women*. "I encourage you to build a strong relationship with herbs."

One note of caution: Many herbs, even those considered generally safe, can cause unwanted side effects in pregnant women. If you're pregnant or suspect that you might be, it's a good idea to avoid using herbs regularly or in medicinal doses unless your obstetrician tells you otherwise. Experts also advise caution while breastfeeding, to ensure a safe supply of breast milk.

Aloe

Aloe barbadensis
Also known as aloes; aloe vera

Regarded as a skin soother since the days of ancient Egypt, this spiky, spiny plant appears in a wide variety of first-aid and hair-care products and cosmetics.

Highly regarded as nature's first line of treatment for skin irritations, minor cuts, and minor burns, aloe's transparent gel effectively hastens wound healing and promotes cell growth and attachment. Aloe shows potential healing qualities for psoriasis and frostbite.

For best results, herbalists recommend snapping off a lower aloe leaf near the center stalk, removing any spines, and then splitting the leaf in half. Scrape the oozing gel directly onto your wound. Fresh gel delivers greater healing power than first-aid products containing aloe.

Do not ingest the leaf. It can cause intense cramping and is a potentially toxic, habit-forming laxative. Aloe may delay deep wound healing, so do not use the gel on any surgical incision.

Angelica

Angelica archangelica

Also known as root of the Holy Ghost; herb of the angel

According to Renaissance folklore, God answered the prayers of a Benedictine monk by revealing angelica as a cure for the Great Plague. Today, this bitter herb appears in European patent medicines, including sedatives, digestive aids, and cramp relievers. Some herbalists believe that angelica promotes circulation and works on congestion, colds, flu, menstrual irregularities, and cramps.

Angelica has a bitter taste that appears to trigger a sensory response in the mouth that can aid digestion and ease gas and stomach cramps. Its roots and leaves are used as a tincture or a tea.

Be aware that angelica looks like hemlock, a deadly poison, so never harvest angelica in the wild. Also, use angelica sparingly and for only short periods of time since prolonged use can cause rashes or sun sensitivity.

Astragalus

Astragalus membranaceous
Also known as huang qi; milk-vetch root

Used for more than 2,000 years by traditional Chinese healers, astragalus has also gained respect among Western herbalists ever since its effects as an immune-system booster came to light.

Herbalists say that astragalus is a natural choice for anyone who might have a weakened immune system, from cold sufferers to cancer patients. Evidence indicates that astragalus helps the body produce protective antibodies and interferon as well as white blood cells. It also contains high amounts of a type of molecule that seems to have anti-cancer qualities. The healing properties are found in the root only.

Astragalus is sold in tincture, tonic, and capsule form. Be patient. It may take a few weeks to show its effects. Astragalus is generally regarded as safe.

Basil

Ocimum basilicum
Also known as sweet basil

A native of India, basil was introduced into Europe during ancient times. In some cultures, basil is regarded as a love token. In others, it is associated with hatred and misfortune.

Now a standard herb in many American kitchens, basil is used medicinally to treat a wide range of conditions, including diarrhea, fever, and jet lag. It may also improve memory.

Basil contains many antiviral compounds. It helps to relieve depression as well.

The leaves contain the medicinal substances. Fresh leaves rubbed on insect bites take away the itch. As an essential oil,

The Name Game

Down in the fields of Texas, wild plants that the locals call milkweeds grow in abundance. But if you ask herbal educator and Texas native Ginger Webb to dig up information about milkweed, she won't be able to help you. "Everything here is called milkweed. Many different plants got called milkweed because they all have a milky sap inside. That name doesn't really tell me anything," Webb says.

Just as one name can be attached to many different plants, one plant can go by many different names. "Someone is talking about coneflower and another person is talking about snakeroot. They are both talking about echinacea," says Webb, the herbal education coordinator for the American Botanical Council in Austin, Texas.

The best way to be accurate when discussing herbs is to use their botanical names, Webb says. The botanical name is the scientific identification botanists give to a plant. No two plants have the same botanical name, so you're guaranteed to get the right herb when you use its official moniker.

Even for the most popular herbs, it's wise to know their proper names. For instance, the widely known term *ginseng* is used to describe three different plants. Two types, *Panax ginseng* (Korean ginseng) and *Panax quinquefolium* (American ginseng), are related. But what people call Siberian ginseng—with the botanical name of *Eleutherococcus senticosus*—isn't a true species of ginseng at all. "Learning the botanical names helps so that when you look up information about a plant, you know you are not getting information about some other plant," Webb notes.

basil is used for nervous exhaustion and mental fatigue. As a tincture, it helps in relieving coughs and bronchitis.

Herbalists advise not taking large amounts of basil tea (several cups per day) for extended periods. Also, the essential oil may irritate the skin if used in a high concentration.

Bearberry

Arctostaphylos uva-ursi

Also known as uva-ursi; bear's grape; mountain box

Marco Polo heard about bearberry's medicinal potential during his journey through Asia. It's unclear if he took this herb back home, but by the 13th century, bearberry was considered an important medicinal herb in Europe. This ground cover was so named because its bright red berries attract bears.

Bearberry is used by herbalists to treat chronic bladder infections by means of an antiseptic contained in the leaves. The leaves also contain antibiotic substances as well as compounds that can help reduce pain in the urinary tract.

Bearberry can be taken as a tincture, as a tea, or in capsules. Herbalists recommend not taking bearberry for more than 2 weeks because its leaves contain tannin, a natural compound that can irritate the stomach. Also, don't use it if you have a kidney disease because the tannin can cause more damage.

Black Cohosh

Cimicifuga racemosa

Also known as black snakeroot; bugbane; rattleroot; rattleweed; squawroot

Derived from the Algonquian word meaning "knobby, rough roots," black cohosh was used by American herbal healers in the 1800s to treat conditions as varied as snakebite, smallpox, and hypochondria.

Today, we know that black cohosh provides a host of nutrients as well as chemicals that help the body produce and use a variety of hormones. Its relaxing and hormone-balancing qualities make it an ideal choice among herbalists for treatment of rheumatoid arthritis, painful or delayed menstruation, menstrual cramps, and hot flashes during menopause.

Select black cohosh in tinctures, capsules, or decoctions that use its root and rhizome, which is a horizontal, underground stem. Don't use the herb for more than 6 months at a time.

Black Haw

Viburnum prunifolium

Also known as stag bush; sweet viburnum; American sloe

Found throughout the eastern and central United States, black haw gained a reputation for preventing miscarriages among Native Americans and pioneers.

Modern herbalists recommend black haw to ease menstrual cramps, ease bleeding after childbirth, and tone down menopausal symptoms. This herb contains four key substances: an aspirin-like compound, a powerful uterine relaxant, a sedative, and steroidlike compounds that may assist the liver in producing hormones.

The bark from its roots, trunk, and branches is best used either boiled down (decocted) into a hot drink or taken as a tincture. People with a history of kidney stones should consult a physician before using black haw since this herb contains substances that can cause kidney stones.

Blue Cohosh

Caulophyllum thalictroides

Also known as papoose root; squawroot

Blue cohosh is one of the oldest-known American herbal remedies. Introduced into medicine in the 1820s, it earned praise for its ability to promote menstruation and to encourage labor.

Blue cohosh contains a chemical that actively stimulates contractions of the uterus and promotes bloodflow to the pelvis. Top herbalists regard blue cohosh as a great choice to help relieve menstrual cramps. This herb also has a reputation for easing rheumatic pain and soothing nervous coughs.

The root and rhizome of blue cohosh can be taken as a

Boost Nutrition with Herbs

"Many herbs are high in vitamins, minerals, and antioxidants," says Jennifer Reid, N.D., a naturopathic physician in Gresham, Oregon.

The bits of garlic clove swimming in your pasta sauce act as a natural antibiotic against infections and help to lower blood pressure and cholesterol. Basil adds flavor to a homemade pizza, but it also improves digestion and mental stimulation.

"Basically, every cooking spice can be considered a good digestive herb that also fights bacteria," says Mindy Green, a founding and professional member of the American Herbalists Guild and director of educational services for the Herb Research Foundation in Boulder, Colorado. "But each herb has its own personality and requires its own special preparation."

Follow these ground rules to reap maximum health benefits from edible herbs.

tincture, as a decoction, or in capsules. The berries are poisonous.

Burdock

Arctium lappa

Also known as beggar's-buttons; clotbur; fox's clote

Burdock possesses a 3,000-year-old reputation for purifying blood and boosting immunity. Seventeenth-century herbalist Nicholas Culpeper declared that burdock root worked wonderfully on bites by "serpents and mad dogs."

Weedy in appearance, with fierce, tenacious burrs, burdock is used by herbalists to treat burns, kidney problems,

Keep a lid on. Herbs' volatile oils, which contain many of their healing properties, can escape into the air if they're left to boil in a pot without a lid, cautions Green.

Activate astragalus. This is one herb that must always be cooked in order for you to benefit from its immunity-boosting and cold-fighting powers. "Even if you bought fresh astragalus and infused it in tea or juice, you would not get the same benefits you would if you cooked it," Green says.

Don't skip supplements. Edible herbs lack the nutritional clout of herbal supplements. "You'd need to take quite a bit to reach a therapeutic dose," says Dr. Reid. "Adding sage to a stew gives flavor, but it probably will not have a noticeable effect on your cold. Taking sage capsules would be much more effective."

rheumatism, and lung infections. The herb contains a compound that both boosts the immune system and shows antidiabetic properties. In addition, burdock's diuretic and mild laxative properties help remove toxins from your body, making it a good choice for psoriasis, eczema, and acne treatment, according to herbal practitioners. Herbalists use the leaves, roots, and seeds of this herb.

Generally regarded as safe, burdock can be used in the form of a tea or tincture or taken in capsules. Its tender leaves can be served raw, steamed, or sautéed.

Calendula

Calendula officinalis
Also known as marybud; pot marigold; gold-bloom

During the Dark Ages, medieval healers advised women to concoct a calendula potion to choose the best suitor. Today, we've left behind superstitious romantic rituals in favor of the practical healing properties that this common garden plant offers. Its orange flower tops and petals contain chemicals that can help reduce inflammation, fight infection, and heal stubborn wounds. Primarily an herb for skin problems, calendula also may show promise in treatments for herpes simplex outbreaks, certain flu viruses, and skin cancer.

Calendula is generally considered to be a safe herb. Forms include teas, tinctures, skin-care creams, and ointments.

Chamomile

Matricaria recutita
Also known as German chamomile

Nicknamed "ground apple" by the ancient Greeks because of its smell, chamomile was also called maythen by the Anglo-Saxons, who regarded it as one of the nine sacred herbs given to the world by the god Woden.

Chamomile has been healing people for more than 2,000 years. It counteracts irritation, soothes upset tummies, shields against ulcers, relaxes muscle spasms, and fights off bacterial and fungal invaders.

A member of the daisy family, it contains a complex collection of compounds that protect and heal the body. One of its chemicals mends torn tissues and heals ulcers. Another kills staphylococcus and streptococcus infections.

You can use this herb in the form of a tea, tincture, or essential oil. If you're allergic to ragweed, asters, and chrysanthemums, however, you're apt to be allergic to chamomile as well. Don't confuse German chamomile with Roman chamomile, which is used in shampoos and cosmetics.

Chasteberry

Vitex agnus-castus

Also known as vitex; monk's pepper

Through the ages, chasteberry was used to quell sexual passion. Today, this highly studied perennial flowering shrub appears to balance hormones during menstruation and menopause. Herbalists say it influences the pituitary gland to stem secretions of the hormone prolactin and allow for a normal menstrual cycle. Chasteberry is the choice for women who experience chronic premenstrual syndrome, menstrual cramps, and menstrual irregularities. It also may be used to aid the body to regain a natural balance after using birth control pills.

The berries are used in teas and tinctures. Be patient. This is a slow-acting herb, so take it regularly for months to reap its benefits. Be aware that chasteberry may counteract the effectiveness of birth control pills.

Comfrey

Symphytum officinale

Also known as boneset; knitback; bruisewort; healing-herb

This herb has been healing wounds since at least the first century B.C. Greek physician Dioscorides proclaimed it as the first completely medicinal herb, unassociated with superstitious practices.

Comfrey has a long history of use, and most of our knowledge comes from tradition. In the past, it was used to reduce inflammation, stimulate the immune system, and ease asthma, ulcers, and lung ailments. Because of safety concerns, however, herbalists no longer recommend it for internal use.

The plant's roots and leaves are used externally—in ointments, poultices, and compresses. Use only dried comfrey, avoiding fresh, young leaves. Do not use on deep or infected wounds; comfrey seems to promote rapid surface healing, which can trap dirt or pus in underlying tissue.

Cramp Bark

Viburnum opulus

Also known as guelder rose; high cranberry; red, rose, or water elder

Birds avoid the bright red berries of the cramp bark bush because they're bitter, but Siberians distill the berries into a soul-warming brew. For more than

700 years, this herb has been prescribed by herbal practitioners to help prevent menstrual cramps, excessive bleeding during menopause, muscle cramps, and pelvic pain.

Nearly identical to black haw, cramp bark is an easy-to-grow shrub with showy white flowers. But cramp bark seems to be a stronger remedy for muscle pain than black haw. That's because cramp bark contains substances that calm the muscle spasms and relax the uterus, which may be how it reduces heavy menstrual bleeding.

The bark is the medicinal part of this herb and is generally regarded as safe.

Dandelion

Taraxacum officinale

Also known as goat's beard; wild chicory; pisseabed; dent de lion

Although today people throughout the world regard this yellow-flowered herb as a troublesome weed, it has been used as a medicinal plant since the times of ancient Greece. Its name probably came from the imagination of a 15th-century surgeon, who compared the shape of the leaves to a lion's tooth, or *dens leonis*.

Dandelion's leaves and roots are used as a diuretic and a liver stimulant. Its roots contain a detoxifier that cleans out various bodily poisons associated with constipation, joint inflammation, acne, fluid retention, and urinary disorders.

Dandelion contains several substances that combine to stimulate bile flow and aid in fat digestion.

Don't use dandelion root without medical approval if you have gallbladder disease.

Dandelion: The Misunderstood Herb

To most people, it's a common weed, and they spend a lot of time and money every year to poison, dig up, and wipe out this useful flower. But throughout history, dandelion has been regarded as a great healer and food source.

You can safely eat every part of the dandelion, says Ellen Evert Hopman, a professional member of the American Herbalists Guild from Amherst, Massachusetts, and author of *Tree Medicine, Tree Magic* and *A Druid's Herbal for the Sacred Earth*. Toss the fresh, edible flowers and leaves into salads or cook the leaves like spinach. A tea made from the root, either fresh or dried, is a good liver medicine. Dandelion flowers have even been used to make wine.

Dong Quai

Angelica sinensis

Also known as dang gui; Chinese angelica

Dong quai, one of the most popular of all Chinese herbs, appears in ancient Chinese medical books dating back to 400 B.C. Revered in Asia as a versatile aid for women's health, dong quai has found use in traditional Chinese medicine for treating allergies, arthritis, nervousness, and high blood pressure.

Herbalists say that dong quai relaxes the uterus, regulates menstruation, reduces hot flashes, reverses vaginal dryness, and clears eczema and psoriasis. Dong quai contains vitamins B_{12} and E and other active compounds, including ferulic acid, which ease menstrual cramps, muscle spasms, and other types of pain. It also contains folate and biotin. These vitamins, along with B_{12}, stimulate the cre-

When harvesting dandelion on your own, choose flowers that lie at least 1,000 feet away from a roadway. Also, use only plants that you absolutely know are free of herbicides and pesticides. When you get home, wash the plants well under running water to remove any clinging dirt.

The leaves taste best in early spring, but you can continue to gather the youngest, most tender shoots throughout the summer. After rinsing, toss with olive oil and lemon juice. If you find the leaves bitter, mix them with lettuce. As you acquire a palate for this backyard delicacy, cut back on the amount of lettuce.

Note: If you have gallbladder disease, do not take dandelion root without medical approval.

ation and development of red blood cells in the bone marrow, which seems to treat a type of anemia associated with menstrual problems.

The herb's root is used in tinctures, teas, and capsules. Herbalists recommend that women stop taking dong quai one week before their menstrual periods and resume taking it at the end of their periods since it can increase blood loss.

Echinacea

Echinacea angustifolia; E. purpurea

Also known as purple coneflower; Kansas or Missouri snakeroot

Echinacea is the world's most researched herb. Its use goes back to the North American Plains Indians, who used it as a remedy more often than any other plant.

Today, echinacea is America's most popular medicinal herb. It is used primarily for colds, flu, infections, slow-healing wounds, and overall immunity boosting.

Echinacea contains many biologically active substances, including some that strengthen the immune system and kill viruses.

The root is used medicinally in tinctures or capsules. Don't use echinacea if you have tuberculosis or an autoimmune condition such as leukosis (a precursor of leukemia), multiple sclerosis, lupus, or any collagen disease. Also, avoid using it if you're allergic to plants in the daisy family, such as marigolds and chamomile.

Eucalyptus

Eucalyptus globulus

Also known as blue gum; fever tree

In the land down under, eucalyptus trees engulf more than three-quarters of the continent. Aborigines and early Australian settlers quenched their thirst by drinking water stored in its roots. The tree was introduced to North America and Europe in the 19th century by the director of the Melbourne Botanical Gardens.

Eucalyptus leaves contain a chemical that herbalists think eases respiratory infections such as bronchitis, sore throats, coughs, fevers, and laryngitis. The aromatic oils of eucalyptus tea spread through the lungs, where they loosen and remove mucus, which can then be cleared out by coughing.

Eucalyptus leaves are brewed into teas, and the essential oil appears in cough drops, nasal inhalers and sprays, sore-muscle rubs, and other preparations. Taking more than 4,000 milligrams a day can cause nausea, vomiting, and diarrhea. Do not use this herb if you have inflammatory disease of the bile ducts or severe liver disease. Do not use the essential oil for more than 2 weeks at a time or apply it to your face. It may irritate your skin if used in a high concentration.

Evening Primrose

Oenothera biennis

Also known as tree primrose; scabbish; cure-all

The Iroquois Indians used evening primrose as a hemorrhoid remedy. The Cherokees drank evening primrose tea as a weight loss tonic and applied the hot root externally for the treatment of hemorrhoids.

Today, both mainstream doctors and herbalists recommend using the oil extracted from the seeds of this nightblossoming herb to ease a wide range of problems. Evening primrose oil helps to lessen some menopausal symptoms as well as chronic inflammatory conditions, such as eczema, hay fever, asthma, and arthritis. Its oil is abundant in essential fatty acids, which help the body to manufacture substances that lower blood pressure, control stomach acids and body temperature, and regulate inflammation. It also shows promise as a fighter against America's top killers, heart disease and cancer.

Evening primrose oil is usually taken in capsule form and is generally regarded as safe.

Fennel

Foeniculum vulgare

Also known as sweet fennel

Ancient Romans believed that serpents sucked the juice of fennel to improve their eyesight. Ancient Greeks regarded fennel as an aid to weight loss. In medieval times, churchgoers chewed fennel seeds to subdue stomach rumblings.

Rich in volatile oils, fennel seeds taste faintly of licorice and are often used to flavor pickles, candies, and breads. Medicinally, the seeds and the fresh stems and bulbs are used to relieve flatulence, aid digestion, regulate appetite, fight infection, heal snakebites, and increase the flow of milk in nursing mothers. Fennel seems to work in the digestive system by soothing the small and large intestines.

Add fennel seeds to food or brew them into teas. Fennel tinctures and capsules are also available. Don't use them medicinally for more than 6 weeks, however, without supervision by a health care practitioner qualified in herbal remedies.

Feverfew

Chrysanthemum parthenium; Tanacetum parthenium
Also known as featherfew; flirtwort; vetter-voo

Seventeenth-century herbalists recommended feverfew as a good herb for getting rid of bad headaches. In the past, women took feverfew to stimulate the expulsion of the placenta after birth and to resolve a host of uterine disorders.

Today, the leaves are used to reduce swelling, relax blood vessels, aid digestion, promote menstruation, and stop headaches. Feverfew may stop throbbing headaches, including migraines, by inhibiting hormones that help to constrict blood vessels. Daily use may help prevent migraines from starting. Scientists theorize that feverfew's active compounds hinder inflammation-inducing agents in the body.

You can chew fresh feverfew leaves or add them to salads. You can infuse them into vinegar or oil as well. Feverfew can also be brewed into a tea or taken freeze-dried in capsules. The capsules must contain at least 0.2 percent parthenolide to be effective. Fresh feverfew leaves can cause mouth sores in sensitive people. Also, avoid using feverfew if you're taking blood-thinning medicines because feverfew can affect clotting rates.

Garlic

Allium sativum

Also known as stinking rose

This humble gray bulb was, and still is, used world-wide by all three classic healing systems: traditional Chinese medicine, traditional European medicine, and Ayurveda. In the first century B.C., Greek physician Dioscorides declared that garlic "clears the arteries and opens the mouths of the veins"—a fact supported by science today.

Garlic helps lower blood cholesterol and blood pressure, prevent blood clots, and improve the overall health of the cardiovascular system. The medicinal source can be found inside garlic cloves, where a sulfur-containing amino acid called alliin resides. When garlic is crushed, alliin converts into allicin, a potent but unstable antibiotic. In addition to its cardiovascular benefits, garlic also combats bacterial and fungal infections. Further, studies suggést that it may help to prevent cancer.

To enjoy the full healing power of garlic, experts advise that you eat raw cloves, but you can also cook garlic, drink it as a maceration (steeped in water or milk overnight), or swallow garlic capsules. You shouldn't use garlic supplements if you're on anticoagulants because garlic can thin your blood and increase bleeding. For the same reasons, don't use garlic before surgery. And don't use it if you're taking hypoglycemic drugs. Finally, women should avoid using fresh garlic while nursing, since it may give the baby gas or indigestion.

Garlic and Bad Breath

There's a reason garlic's nickname is the "stinking rose." Fresh garlic contains sulfur compounds, which deliver that characteristic pungent odor, explains Jennifer Reid, N.D., a naturopathic physician in Gresham, Oregon.

Among medicinal herbs, garlic has been revered for centuries by Greek and Roman healers. In the past 2 decades, more than 1,000 research studies have been published about garlic's role as a natural antibiotic, bacteria fighter, and cholesterol reducer. Specifically, its sulfur-scented healing compound, called allicin, is activated whenever garlic cloves are crushed, cut, or chewed. Allicin is also released when enteric-coated garlic products, such as capsules, are broken down in the intestines.

So if you love garlic, what can you do to camouflage its odor? You could convince your close friends to eat garlic with you. Or you could end a garlic-laden meal by nibbling parsley. Fresh parsley sprigs contain a high level of chlorophyll, and chlorophyll is the key ingredient in many breath fresheners, explains Dr. Reid.

You can also prevent bad breath by taking enteric-coated garlic products or organic odorless garlic powder capsules in lieu of the clove itself, but garlic's stubborn odor will permeate through your skin whenever you sweat, says Dr. Reid.

Ginger

Zingiber officinale

Also known as Jamaican ginger; African ginger; Cochin ginger

Emperor Shen Nung immortalized ginger's healing powers in the *Pen Tsao Ching (The Classic Book of Herbs)* in 3000 B.C., and it is still widely used in China today.

Ginger surpasses all other herbs when it comes to suppressing the queasiness of motion sickness, and studies show that it also works better than the active ingredient in over-the-counter drugs like Dramamine. Ginger settles upset stomachs, relieves vomiting, and eases gas pain and diarrhea by stimulating saliva flow and digestive activity. Its gingerols and shogaols are considered effective antinausea workhorses.

Take fresh or dried gingerroot in teas, tinctures, or capsules, or add it to food dishes. Since ginger may increase bile secretion, anyone with gallstones should check with a health care practitioner qualified in herbal remedies before using the dried root in therapeutic amounts. Avoid it if you have ulcers since it will overstimulate the stomach, herbalists say.

Ginkgo

Ginkgo biloba

Also known as maidenhair tree

The seeds of the ginkgo tree have been used as both food and medicine for thousands of years, but today we use the leaves of the plant.

Ginkgo is considered a good anti-aging herb because it benefits organs usually diminished by time: the eyes, brain, blood vessels, and cardiovascular system.

Scientists have learned that concentrated ginkgolide, a substance extracted from the leaves, sharpens memory, boosts concentration, reduces anxiety, lessens the symptoms of Alzheimer's disease, lowers blood pressure, relieves headaches, and improves a litany of circulation problems.

Ginkgo also contains derivatives of a compound called terpene, which acts as a bodyguard for the brain, protecting against blood clots and nerve damage. Ginkgo's flavonoids help stop the action of damaging free radicals.

Purchase ginkgo extracts that contain standardized amounts of ginkgolide for maximum benefits. Experts suggest products whose labels say "24/6," which means the product contains 24 percent glycosides and 6 percent terpenes. Diarrhea, vomiting, and dermatitis may occur if you take more than 240 milligrams of concentrated ginkgo daily. The usual daily dose is 120 milligrams.

Avoid taking ginkgo with antidepressant MAO inhibitor drugs such as phenelzine sulfate (Nardil) or tranylcypromine (Parnate), aspirin or other nonsteroidal anti-inflammatory medications, or blood-thinning medications such as warfarin (Coumadin).

Ginseng

Panax ginseng (Korean ginseng); P. quinquefolium (American ginseng)

Also known as sang; root of life; a dose of immortality

For thousands of years, ginseng has had a nearly mythical reputation as a cure-all herb. Explorer Marco Polo wrote of this prized wonder drug, and Native Americans used American ginseng, hoping it would help with menstrual problems, headaches, exhaustion, fever, colic, vomiting, and earaches.

Today, many Asians use ginseng to renew and enhance sexual desire and ease difficult childbirth.

Another kind of ginseng, Siberian (*Eleutherococcus senticosus*), is not a true form of ginseng, but it shares certain properties with the Korean and American herbs.

Science hasn't completely proven that ginseng helps with all of those conditions, but scientists have discovered that the root contains at least 18 different hormonelike substances. These fight stress and fatigue, protect the liver, and prevent memory loss. This herb is often used to relieve stress-related hot flashes at menopause.

The root can be chewed or made into a tea. Ginseng is also available in capsules, tablets, and liquid extracts. Avoid it while consuming caffeine or other stimulants because it may cause irritability. Don't take it if you have high blood pressure.

Goldenseal

Hydrastis canadensis

Also known as orange root; yellow root; jaundice root; eye balm

Native to North America, goldenseal was used extensively by Native Americans as a clothing dye and a war paint as well as a remedy. The wrinkled, chrome-yellow root was used by the Cherokee to soothe inflammation and spark appetite. The Iroquois washed sore eyes with it. The Micmac applied goldenseal to chapped lips.

Although goldenseal is the third-best-selling herb in the United States, there has been little scientific study of its usefulness. Nevertheless, many herbalists depend on goldenseal to alleviate sinus infections, colds and flu, laryngitis, sore throats, mouth sores, colitis, gastritis, ear-

Why Are Some Herbs So Expensive?

One great thing about herbs: They're a lot cheaper than visits to the doctor or prescription medications, right? Unfortunately, that isn't necessarily so. If you haven't taken a stroll down the herb aisle in a health food store lately, be prepared for sticker shock.

As with many products, supply and demand dictate the price, says Jennifer Brett, N.D., a naturopathic physician in Stratford, Connecticut. For instance, when St. John's wort shot up in popularity in 1997, manufacturers scrambled to harvest all they could, so the supply quickly dwin-

aches, and vaginal infections. Goldenseal root contains substances that act as natural antibiotics, inflammation stoppers, uterine tonics, and digestive helpers.

Herbalists use the roots in teas, tinctures, capsules, eyewashes, gargles, ear drops, douches, and disinfectant salves. Goldenseal is safe when used topically, but do not use it internally for more than 3 weeks since it may irritate your mucous membranes. Also, don't use goldenseal if you have high blood pressure.

Green Tea

Camellia sinensis

Also known, in China, as cha

Green tea has been used in China for more than 5,000 years, and it has become so common in our own culture that you may overlook its important role as a medicinal herb.

died. No new St. John's wort could be collected until it re-
grew, which took another growth cycle. This made the
price per capsule rise dramatically.

Sometimes the demand actually endangers a species,
driving prices up even more. Goldenseal has become an en-
dangered plant in several states, thanks to its popularity.
Demand always exceeds the supply, which is why you pay
top dollar for this herb. Good-quality goldenseal roots sell
at $20 per pound—a steep price when most other plants
are usually sold for $1 to $2 per pound, Dr. Brett notes.

Green tea is amazingly versatile. It contains polyphenols,
or catechins, which protect your heart by lowering cholesterol levels and improving the way your body metabolizes
fats. These substances also fight bacterial invaders. They
may help guard against cancer by collecting free radicals
that can damage cells and push them toward uncontrolled
growth. Green tea contains fluoride, so it can lessen the risk
of tooth decay. It is also used to treat insect bites.

People with asthma benefit from drinking green tea because it contains a substance, a close cousin of caffeine,
that opens up bronchial tubes.

Green tea leaves are primarily brewed to drink, but you
can also use them to make an effective poultice or compress.

People with irregular heartbeats should limit their intake to no more than two cups of green tea daily because
the caffeinelike alkaloids can speed up heart rates. Its
bitter taste stimulates gastric acid production, so green tea
should be consumed in limited amounts by those with
stomach ulcers.

Immunity-Enhancing Herbal Soup

Try this easy soup to help stop a cold in its tracks, fend off the flu, or banish sluggish, achy, or stressed-out feelings. Although the chicken broth masks the taste of the medicinal herbs, rest assured that they'll still be working, says herbalist Rosemary Gladstar, director of the Sage Mountain Herbal Education Center in East Barre, Vermont. (Vegetarians can replace the chicken broth with miso soup.)

  2 cans (16 ounces each) chicken broth
  ¾ cup water
  1 red onion, chopped
  1 red bell pepper, thinly sliced
  1 teaspoon lemon juice
  2 cloves garlic, minced
  1 slice fresh astragalus
  1 tablespoon fresh or dried burdock root (see note)
  1 tablespoon fresh or dried dandelion root (see note)
  1 tablespoon dried Siberian ginseng
  ¼ teaspoon fresh or dried thyme
  2 pinches ground red pepper

In a 3-quart saucepan, mix the broth, water, onion, bell pepper, lemon juice, garlic, astragalus, burdock root, dandelion root, ginseng, thyme, and ground red pepper. Bring to a boil. Cover, reduce the heat to low, and simmer for 15 minutes. Remove and discard the astragalus, dried burdock, and dried dandelion.

Note: If using fresh burdock and dandelion roots, slice thinly and mix directly into the soup. If using dried burdock and dandelion, place them in a mesh bag for easy removal.

Hawthorn

Crataegus oxycantha; C. laevigata; C. monogyna

Also known as May blossom; whitethorn; haw

In the past, this fast-growing hedge and ornamental shrub was used for weak stomachs, edema, and as a first-aid tool to draw splinters. By the early 1900s, however, herbal doctors began prescribing hawthorn for cardiac weakness, heart pain, and irregular heartbeats.

Now hawthorn's red berries, white flowers, and leaves are recognized by herbalists as useful for long-term cardiovascular health. They contain compounds that dilate arteries and lower blood pressure when taken for at least 6 months. Hawthorn also stimulates circulation and helps deliver oxygen to the heart.

Hawthorn is primarily taken as a tea but also may be used as a tincture. Have your doctor monitor your heart health if you take hawthorn regularly for more than 3 weeks. In some instances, you may need lower doses of other medicines, such as drugs for high blood pressure. If you have heart valve problems that cause low blood pressure, don't use hawthorn without a physician's supervision.

Kava Kava

Piper methysticum

Also known as intoxicating pepper

Native to tropical forests, kava kava is a staple at some Polynesian religious rites, during which participants drink it as a fermented liquor. Kava kava can relax you and evoke restful sleep without numbing your mind or leaving you with a hangover.

Kava kava belongs to a class of herbs called nervines, which seem to nudge into action the part of the nervous system that helps us to relax. It is effective against tension headaches, anxiety, insomnia, and cramps caused by endometriosis. The dried root of kava kava reduces muscle spasms, soothes pain, and heightens your sense of well-being.

Sometimes used as a tea, kava kava is also available in tinctures and capsules. Do not exceed the recommended doses. Because the herb is a mild sedative and muscle relaxant, never take it with alcohol or barbiturates, and use caution when driving or operating equipment.

Lady's-Mantle

Alchemilla vulgaris
Also known as ladies mantle; lion's foot; bear's foot

Highly astringent and rich in tannins, lady's-mantle was used to heal wounds sustained in battle during the 15th and 16th centuries. As its name implies, this herb with gray-green leaves and lacy blooms is considered a valuable gynecological remedy as well.

Its astringent properties make it an excellent herb for normalizing bleeding from heavy periods or fibroid tumors. It also improves uterine tone, subdues menopausal hot flashes, and soothes mild menstrual aches and pains.

In addition, its leaves and flowers help close and heal wounds. When they're taken internally, they help relieve bleeding and diarrhea.

Use the leaves, stems, and flowers of lady's-mantle internally in a tea or tincture or externally as an herbal wash or poultice. The herb is generally considered safe.

Lavender

Lavandula officinalis; L. angustifolia; L. vera

Also known as true lavender; garden lavender

Ancient Greeks imported lavender from Syria because of its fragrance, which freshened rooms, perfumes, and baths.

Today, lavender is a key ingredient in smelling salts.

The fragrant, volatile oil in its blossoms contains more than 100 chemical compounds that calm the central nervous system. As a tea, it tastes soapy, so you may want to add honey. Lavender is also taken as a tincture or used externally as an essential oil in baths, facial steams, and massage oils. It is generally considered to be safe.

Lemon Balm

Melissa officinalis

Also known as sweet balm; balm; melissa

Lemon balm has been linked with bees since ancient times; in fact, its botanical name, *Melissa*, comes from the Greek word for honeybee. Up until the 18th century, lemon balm was thought to renew youth.

Today, its fuzzy, citrus-scented leaves are used to calm tension, raise the spirits, and relieve depression, insomnia, nervousness, and tension headaches. Since it relieves gas, it can tame digestive discomfort, especially when stress is the cause. It contains oils that are full of terpenes, substances that have antiviral properties and may help to fight herpes outbreaks. Women also rely on lemon balm to relax uterine spasms that cause painful periods.

Lemon balm is usually taken as a tea or used in ointments or as a calming bath. It's considered to be a safe herb.

Licorice

Glycyrrhiza glabra

Also known as sweet wood

Used as medicine for more than 2,500 years and nick-named the "great detoxifier" in China, licorice is thought to drive poisons from the body. In 17th-century England, licorice was boiled with figs to silence coughs and ease chest pains.

The root of this versatile herb, sometimes called the grandfather of herbs, is found in many herbal formulas for women because it contains estrogen-like compounds. This makes it valuable for regulating hormones at menopause. In addition, licorice contains a compound called glycyrrhizin, which is 50 times sweeter than sugar. It also has substances that help fight inflammation, allergies, and arthritis.

To treat arthritis and allergic conditions, use it in a tincture; for asthma and bronchitis, take it in a syrup, herbalists recommend. For ulcers, drink it as a decoction to reduce stomach acid. Never use licorice if you have diabetes, high blood pressure, a heart condition, liver or kidney disorders, or low potassium levels. And don't use it for more than 4 to 6 weeks.

Marshmallow

Althaea officinalis

Also known as cheeses

Marshmallow's slippery, sweet main ingredient was used for thousands of years as a soothing cure for coughs, sore throats, wheezing, and irritated skin. It gained a reputation as a tasty treat only a few centuries ago, when a spongy mix of sugar, egg whites, and ground marshmallow root, called *pate de guimauve*, became a trendy royal dessert

Is Licorice Candy Effective?

That flexible black candy stick you love munching on shares its name and sweet taste with a medicinal plant, but nothing else. Licorice candy contains mostly corn syrup, sugar, and artificial flavoring. The medicinal herb form of licorice contains glycyrrhizin, a bacteria-killing, nonsugar sweetener.

Licorice is well-regarded among herbalists for its versatility in treating many conditions. Licorice tea soothes the mucous membranes, making it a preferred choice for coughs, asthma, and sore throats, says Rosita Arvigo, a master herbalist, doctor of naprapathy (a form of chiropractic), author of *Rainforest Remedies*, and director of the Ix Chel Tropical Research Foundation in Belize, Central America. For the best medicinal form, select deglycyrrhizinated licorice extracts (DGLE).

If you enjoy licorice candy but want medicinal benefits, too, try the fresh (and genuine) licorice sticks available in health food stores. You'll enjoy their sweet taste, and they may clear up any congestion that has you down.

Keep in mind that ingesting excessive amounts of licorice can cause water retention, headaches, or high blood pressure from potassium loss. Do not use licorice for more than 4 to 6 weeks, and avoid it if you have diabetes, high blood pressure, or a heart, liver, or kidney condition.

in Europe. Unfortunately, modern-day marshmallow candy lacks any real marshmallow root.

Researchers have discovered why this pretty marsh-dwelling plant heals wounded skin and soothes mucous membranes. The root contains high amounts of a slippery, indigestible complex sugar, called mucilage, that coats, cools, and moisturizes wounded, inflamed tissues from the throat to the intestines to the urinary tract. Herbalists also use marshmallow root for mouth sores, gastritis, peptic ulcers, irritating coughs, varicose veins, and burns.

Take marshmallow as a cold or hot tea or use it as a poultice of mashed roots. Because it will coat the linings of your digestive tract, keep in mind that marshmallow may slow absorption of other medications taken at the same time.

Milk Thistle

Silybum marianum

Also known as Mary thistle; Marian thistle; lady's thistle

The famous English herbalist known only as Gerald described milk thistle as "the best remedy that grows, against all melancholy diseases." In the Middle Ages, melancholy was associated with any liver- or bile-related illness.

Herbalists recommend this herb's seeds for increasing the secretion and flow of bile from the liver and gallbladder. Milk thistle's active ingredient, silymarin, is one of the strongest liver protectors known. Scientists have learned that the compound improves cirrhosis, hepatitis, and liver damage caused by toxic chemicals. As an antioxidant, it may be 10 times stronger than vitamin E.

Take milk thistle in the form of tea, capsules, tablets, and tinctures. It's considered to be a safe herb.

Motherwort

Leonurus cardiaca

Also known as mother herb; heart heal; lion's tail; lion's ear

Motherwort was once regarded as a powerful defender against wicked spirits, and it was used for thousands of years to dispel doldrums and anxiety. The ancient Chinese believed motherwort could lengthen life. In the past, its dull green leaves and purplish blooms were called upon to induce menstruation and alleviate fainting.

Motherwort's leaves and flowers contain substances that promote menstrual bleeding. The herb also contains mild sedatives and relaxants that may temporarily lower blood pressure. Herbalists believe these compounds soothe the stress of premenstrual tension and menopausal hot flashes, restore cardiac health, and tone down a rapid heartbeat brought on by anxiety.

Use motherwort as a tea or tincture. For tension relief, it may take about 15 minutes before you feel the effects. It is generally regarded as safe.

Mullein

Verbascum thapsus

Also known as candlewick; velvet dock; Arron's rod; Peter's staff

Mullein's tall stems, which are covered in fine down, were once burned as tapers in funeral processions. Greek physician Dioscorides used the herb for scorpion stings, eye problems, and toothaches.

Today herbalists use mullein's velvety leaves and flowers to help treat bronchitis, colds and flu, coughs, earaches, emphysema, and laryngitis. It works for respiratory complaints because it helps bring up sticky phlegm, soothes sore throats, fights bacterial invaders, and stops muscle spasms that trigger coughs. It also contains compounds that inhibit flu viruses.

Use mullein in teas, tinctures, mouthwashes, and syrups. It is generally regarded as safe.

Herb and Drug Interactions

Even though herbs can be safer than over-the-counter or prescription drugs, they should be regarded as medicine. Don't take herbs and over-the-counter medications at the same time for the same condition. And inform your doctor of any herbs you take, especially if you're on prescription medicines.

Type of Drug

Anti-allergy drugs such as diphenhydramine (Benadryl), hydroxyzine (Vistaril), and astemizole (Hismanal)

Antidepressant drugs such as fluoxetine (Prozac), amitriptyline (Elavil), and imipramine (Trofranil)

Blood pressure medicines such as enalapril (Vaseretic) and prazosin (Minizide)

Cardiac glycosides, which include digitalis medications, such as digoxin (Lanoxin)

Diuretics, such as furosemide (Lasix) and indapamide (Lozol)

Hypnotic and mild sedative drugs, such as diazepam (Valium), flurazepam, and alprazolam (Xanax)

Laxative drugs, such as docusate sodium (Colace) and psyllium (Metamucil), and polycarbophil (FiberCon)

Not all herb–drug interactions are known. This table offers information on some potential interactions between herbs and medications for common conditions, based on medical research.

Type of Herb	Possible Effects If Combined
Sedative herbs such as skullcap, passionflower, and valerian	Drowsiness caused by antihistamine drugs may increase
Sedative herbs such as skullcap, passionflower, and valerian	Sedative side effects of the drug may increase
Herbs with ingredients that may raise blood pressure, such as licorice	The drug's effects may lessen
Diuretic herbs and herbs with ingredients that may lower blood pressure, such as garlic and hawthorn	The drug's effects may be increased or altered
Herbs with ingredients that can affect the cardiovascular system, such as coltsfoot, motherwort, hawthorn, and goldenseal	The drug's effects may increase
Diuretic herbs such as dandelion, uva-ursi, buchu, and cornsilk	Diuretic effects may be much stronger, with a risk of abnormally low potassium levels
Sedative herbs such as skullcap, passionflower, and valerian	The drug's sedative effect may increase
Laxative herbs such as aloe, cascara sagrada, plantain, rhubarb, senna, and yellow dock	The drug's effects may increase

Nettle

Urtica dioica

Also known as stinging nettle; wild spinach

Historically, Europeans used nettle gargles to ease sore, swollen throats and prepared nettle drinks to expel kidney stones by increasing urination. Native Americans used nettle to treat ills as varied as coughs, colds, epilepsy, gout, stomachaches, insanity, and even hair loss. Nineteenth-century Americans used nettle tea to treat diarrhea, dysentery, and hemorrhoids.

Today's herbalists are more judicious and realistic. They use nettle as a diuretic as well as an astringent to stop nosebleeds, wound bleeding, and heavy menstrual flow. Some herbalists believe it may also alleviate sinus problems, allergies, and hay fever. Used externally, nettle soothes insect bites and stings as well as burns.

Take this herb as a tea, as a tincture, or freeze-dried in capsules. It can also be used as a compress. Some people's allergy symptoms may worsen, rather than improve, after using nettle, so medical experts advise taking no more than one dose a day for the first few days.

Oatstraw

Avena sativa

Also known as wild oats

Oats have been cultivated as a food since at least 100 B.C. The straw, made into a tea, was used as a folk remedy for nervous exhaustion and sleeplessness. Traditionally, a good soak in an oatstraw bath was said to relieve arthritis and rheumatism.

Today, oatstraw is considered an excellent tonic for the whole body. It treats tension headaches, insomnia, nervous exhaustion, and physical fatigue. Oatstraw contains calcium and silicic acid (a component of silica), reportedly making this herb a good tonic for hair, nails, and bones.

Oat's stems, leaves, and husks are used in teas and tinctures or in healing washes for skin conditions. Oatstraw contains the grain protein gluten, so don't ingest it if you have gluten intolerance (celiac disease).

Partridgeberry

Mitchella repens

Also known as squaw vine; deer berry; mountain tea; winter clover; hive vine

From the Cherokee to the Iroquois, Native American women turned to this low-growing herb to alleviate menstrual cramps and soothe sore nipples while nursing.

Today this evergreen with shiny leaves and brilliant red berries is still considered among the best remedies for bringing on missed menstrual periods, easing cramps, and lightening heavy menstrual flow.

The leaves, stems, and berries are used in teas and tinctures. Partridgeberry is generally considered safe.

Passionflower

Passiflora incarnata

Also known as maypop; passion-vine; Holy Trinity flower

The exotic and intricate flowers of this plant reminded Spanish explorers and missionaries of the crown of thorns of Christ's passion. Hence its name, which refers to spiritual suffering, not sexual passion.

Passionflower grows wild in the southern United States. Its flowers, leaves, and vine contain sedatives, so it's used as a remedy for rattled nerves and for inducing sleep when anxiety or the insomnia of menopause interrupts nighttime rest. It may also help calm other conditions, such as hot flashes, abdominal pain, headaches, and high blood pressure, when they're related to stress.

Passionflower is usually taken as a tea or tincture. It's generally regarded as safe.

Peppermint

Mentha piperita

Also known as field mint

Across the globe and throughout the centuries, peppermint has earned a reputation as a stomach-soothing, gas-repressing, nausea-reversing herb. In medieval Europe, after-dinner peppermint jellies aided in digestion. Arabs finished dinners with a mint tea. The Cherokee used peppermint to treat vomiting, colic, and gas.

Today, peppermint's stature among herbalists as a medicinal herb to treat nausea, vomiting, indigestion, flatulence, hiccups, and stomach muscle spasms remains unchallenged. Peppermint leaves contain menthol-rich volatile oils, which act as a mild anesthetic to the stomach wall. They also contain tannins and bitters, which may kill many kinds of microorganisms and boost mental alertness. Peppermint eases anxiety and tension as well.

If using fresh peppermint, crush the leaves first. Otherwise, take this herb as a tea or tincture. It's generally regarded as a safe herb.

Red Clover

Trifolium pratense

Also known as purple clover; meadow trefoil

Long, long ago, red clover was used strictly as fodder crop for cattle. Then, in medieval times, Christians associated this three-leafed grass with the Trinity. The Chinese relied on red clover's sap as a remedy for colds and influenza. Native Americans used the herb to treat menopausal symptoms.

Red clover blossoms contain estrogen-like substances that can help make the menstrual cycle more regular, enhance fertility, and balance hormones at menopause. Its flowers also contain calcium, magnesium, potassium, and vitamins B and C. They're used internally as a cleanser for skin complaints as well as a medicine for coughs and bronchitis.

This herb is primarily used in teas, tinctures, and compresses.

Rosemary

Rosmarinus officinalis

Also known as incensier

A symbol for remembrance, rosemary is a native Mediterranean shrub that was reputedly first grown in England in the 14th century by Philippa of Hainault, wife of Edward III.

A relative of mint, rosemary is an ideal choice to counter exhaustion, weakness, jet lag, and breast pain. Herbalists think that rosemary may help ease breast pain by acting as a drying agent to fluid-filled cysts. Plus, it helps balance out-of-whack hormones. According to

Herbs to Go

In the top drawer of Sharleen Andrews-Miller's desk, you'll find a pint jar filled to the brim with herbal goodies. It's a mini-kit of ingredients that can treat just about anything.

Andrews-Miller, a faculty member at the National College of Naturopathic Medicine in Portland, Oregon, singled out what she considers the most versatile herbs to have on hand. You should replenish the kit with new material once a year.

- Mason jar or sealed bag—for storing your items and to use for teas
- Small washcloth or sterile gauze pads—for soaks
- Pair of tweezers—always a handy tool
- A few adhesive bandages—for covering cuts and scratches
- Chamomile tea bags in a sealed plastic bag—drink tea for upset stomach and stress relief; apply wet bags to cuts as an antiseptic

herbalists, it's fortified with more than a dozen antioxidants, which mop up free radicals and help prevent aging in cells. It also contains a half-dozen compounds that reportedly prevent the breakdown of a brain chemical that plays a vital role in cognition and reasoning. People with Alzheimer's disease often have a deficit of this chemical.

Rosemary essential oil is popular among aromatherapists for treating mild depression. It contains a compound that is believed to stimulate the central nervous system.

The leaves and stems are used in teas, tinctures, and essential oils. Rosemary may cause excessive menstrual bleeding. Avoid rosemary essential oil if you have epilepsy or hypertension.

- Peppermint tea bags in a sealed plastic bag—drink tea for upset stomach; soak rag in tea and lay on forehead for headache; inhale tea vapors for sinus congestion
- Crystallized ginger—pop a piece in your mouth for nausea
- Rescue Remedy—for trauma and anxiety, place four drops of this Bach flower essence under your tongue
- Lavender essential oil—to lift your mood, inhale the vapors; place oil on a wet washcloth and lay over aching muscles, cuts, insect bites, or sunburn; dab on your temples with your finger for a headache
- Witch hazel pads—for quick wound washes
- Echinacea tincture—put in a spray bottle and spray in your throat when you feel a cold or sore throat coming on; use topically as an antiseptic

St. John's Wort

Hypericum perforatum

Also known as hypericum; St.-Joan's-wort

Known as a wound healer since 500 B.C., this medicinal herb was gathered and burned annually by European peasants on June 24, St. John's Day, to stave off goblins and devils. Its yellow flowers, which release crimson juice when crushed, became a symbol of the blood of St. John the Baptist.

This weedy-looking herb contains at least three key medicinal substances. One of them, hypericin, protects the brain's serotonin, the feel-good chemical. Taken internally, St. John's wort delivers a sedative and pain-reducing effect, making it an ideal choice among herbal healers to treat depression, anxiety, and tension. As a lotion, it helps heal bruises, varicose veins, and sunburn, possibly because it's an anti-inflammatory. When using it for depression, you should buy St. John's wort that contains standardized levels of hypericin—0.3 percent—for best results. It may take 2 to 6 weeks to take effect.

You can use the leaves, stems, and flowers in tea, tincture, powder, capsules, and tablets. Reserve the oil for external use. Be aware that this herb may cause sun sensitivity. Also, avoid taking it with other antidepressants unless you have your doctor's approval.

Skullcap

Scutellaria laterifolia

Also known as mad-dog weed; helmet flower

First used by Native Americans for rabies and menstrual problems, this herb, with its dish-shaped seedpods and delicate blue flowers, is now well-respected as a tonic that nourishes and revitalizes the nervous system.

Skullcap contains minerals (including calcium, iron, potassium, and magnesium) that help you deal with stress, tension headaches, anxiety, exhaustion, and depression. A mild "lullaby herb," skullcap promotes sound sleep without leaving you feeling groggy in the morning. It also eases the moodiness of premenstrual syndrome and severe mood changes during menopause.

Use skullcap's leaves and flowers in teas and tinctures. Although it's generally considered to be safe, do not confuse this herb with Chinese skullcap (*S. baicalensis*), which has totally different properties.

Slippery Elm

Ulmus fulva

Also known as sweet elm; moose elm; Indian elm

Before Dutch elm disease wiped out many of North America's mature trees, people used slippery elm's sweet-tasting inner bark to relieve many ailments—from diarrhea and rheumatism to coughs and ulcers.

Today, herbalists use slippery elm to treat inflammations, such as those that come with bladder infections, diarrhea, peptic ulcers, coughs, colitis, and acid stomach. You can apply homemade paste or gel to wounds or inflamed skin. You can also use the gel to restore vaginal lubrication during menopause. Herbalists say that it's the mucilage in slippery elm bark that helps with inflammation.

The inner bark of slippery elm is made into beverages and healing poultices. This herb is generally considered safe.

Valerian

Valeriana officinalis

Also known as all heal; moon root; great wild valerian

This showy plant with feathery pink blooms possesses such awful-smelling roots that the Greek physician Dioscorides nicknamed it "phu." But smelly or not, valerian has been used as a tranquilizer and anti-insomnia remedy for more than 1,000 years.

Valerian root reduces the time it takes to doze, lessens middle-of-the-night awakenings, and helps you wake up clearheaded. It also relaxes tense nerves and muscles, making it a natural choice for mood swings and menstrual cramps. Its compounds attach to the same brain receptors as tranquilizers like diazepam (Valium), but with milder effects and without the risk of addiction or dependence. Valerian also contains alkaloids that help lower blood pressure.

Take valerian root in teas, tinctures, tablets, or capsules. Do not take valerian with other sleep-enhancing or mood-controlling medications, such as Valium or amitriptyline (Elavil), since it can increase the effects of those drugs. Also, stop using it if you find yourself feeling stimulated, rather than calmed, by it. In some people, it may cause heart palpitations or nervousness.

Yarrow

Achillea millefolium
Also known as nosebleed; millefoil

Yarrow's Latin name comes from the ancient Greek hero Achilles. Its folk name, "nosebleed," refers to its ability to stop bleeding.

Yarrow, with its delicate white flowers and feathery green leaves, contains more than 120 compounds. It is used to reduce fevers, stop inflammation, control heavy menstrual flow, cool hot flashes, heal bladder infections, and relieve colds, flu, coughs, and sore throats. It's also used as a wash or a poultice to stop bleeding and heal wounds and in hot herbal baths to lessen menstrual cramps.

Take yarrow internally as a hot or cold tea, as a tincture, or in capsules. In rare instances, handling its flowers can cause a skin rash.

Yellow Dock

Rumex crispus
Also known as curly dock; narrow-leaved dock

Depending on your point of view, yellow dock is vilified as a stubborn, unruly common weed or credited as a tonic for the bowels, liver, and skin. This long, golden-hued taproot first sprouted in Europe. It was brought to America by colonists.

Herbalists believe prolonged use of yellow dock lessens the effect of chronic skin problems such as acne, eczema, psoriasis, and rashes. The minerals in this herb give a boost to women who feel tired all the time and offer relief as a gentle laxative. Yellow dock contains thiamin, iron, and vitamin C, plus compounds that stimulate bile production and nudge a sluggish liver, according to herb practitioners.

Yellow dock is best taken as a tea or tincture before meals if you want to absorb its nutrients and at bedtime for overnight constipation relief. It's also available in capsules. Yellow dock contains substances that may cause kidney stones, so consult a physician first before using it if you have a history of kidney stones.

PART THREE

Herbs for Body and Soul

The Serenity Herbs

Take 5 minutes and say a prayer for yourself."
That's the advice of herbalist Kathleen Gould when she teaches her students about soothing teas. As masters of the Japanese tea ceremony have known for centuries, making tea involves much more than knowing how many teaspoons to use and how long to let the leaves steep. The making and drinking of an herbal tea should be a relaxing ritual.

"I always try to get my students to do some kind of ceremony," says Gould, a professional member of the American Herbalists Guild and director of the Herb Corner, an herbal teaching school in Indialantic, Florida.

Using herbs to relax and get rid of stress should be more than just taking medicine. It should be part of a rite that celebrates you. "If you are under chronic stress, you never get a break. It is okay to do something for yourself," Gould says.

Many herbs contain substances that help bring on tranquillity and dissipate tension, and they have long been used to soothe away the stresses and strains that most of us undergo in our daily lives. But chemicals and compounds aren't the whole story. The process—the way you use herbs to calm, soothe, and relax—plays a major role in how they work.

Whether you're boiling water for tea, drawing a bath, or massaging your feet with herbal oil, there is something so soothing and peaceful in the act that it can be pure magic. "When you slow down enough to do this for yourself, you'll automatically start feeling a lot better," says Gail Ulrich, an herbalist, director of the Blazing Star Herbal School in Shelburne Falls, Massachusetts, and author of *Herbs to Boost Immunity*.

Which herbs offer solace from a hectic world? Following are some well-known plants that are recommended by herbalists to help you calm down and relax.

Chamomile. In the 19th century, chamomile was used to treat the "nervousness" that sometimes accompanied a menstrual cycle. It's usually taken as a tea.

Lavender. The volatile oil in lavender, which contains more than 100 chemical compounds, calms the nervous system. It can be taken in a tea or tincture or used externally in baths and massage oils.

Lemon balm. Lemon balm calms tension, raises spirits, and relieves depression, insomnia, nervousness, and tension headaches. It's also known to pacify an upset stomach caused by stress. Lemon balm is usually used in tea or baths.

Oatstraw. This is a popular choice to allay tension headaches, insomnia, and nervous exhaustion. Oatstraw is mainly used as a tea and tincture.

Passionflower. This herb contains chemicals shown in laboratory studies to have sedating effects. It's often used to help bring on sleep and to ease the stress of premenstrual syndrome. Take it as a tea or tincture.

Skullcap. Thought to nourish the nervous system, this herb helps in times of stress. It also aids tension headaches, anxiety, depression, and exhaustion. It is used as a tea or tincture.

To use these serenity herbs correctly, create an accompanying serene atmosphere. All the lemon balm in the world won't calm you down if you are trying to feed the kids, open the mail, and do the dishes—all while the phone rings incessantly and the evening news blares from the TV.

Here's how to set the mood.

- Take your time. Whatever you are doing, don't rush it. Make sure you give yourself and the herb royal treatment. Celebrate each step of the process, even if it is something as simple as boiling the water, letting the herb steep, and straining the tea.
- Turn off the TV. Unplug the phone. Get rid of distractions.
- Light some candles. Play some soft music. Establish a relaxing ambience.
- Practice deep, slow breathing. This will help you relax and enjoy your herbal remedies.

Recipes for Relaxation

While tinctures, capsules, and teas of each individual serenity herb will help, there are many ways to mix and match them to create a wonderful soothing blend. Herbalists have devised many interesting and even fun ways to enjoy these calming herbs. Here's how you can use them, too.

Brew a calming cup. Sip a cup of this tea when you need to relax and wind down, advises Jennifer Reid, N.D., a naturopathic physician in Gresham, Oregon. It combines several of the soothing serenity herbs. Mix 3 ounces of dried lemon balm, 1½ ounces of dried oatstraw, 1½

THE HERBAL KITCHEN

Insomnia Tea

At one time or another, we all have trouble getting to sleep, so every good herbalist has an insomnia tea recipe, says Shez Ward, an herbalist in Norfolk, England, and a member of the Royal Horticultural Society.

The following recipe, crafted by Ward, combines valerian, which is often recommended for insomnia, with passionflower and skullcap, which are used to relax and soothe.

Brew this tea about 2 hours before you go to bed. It takes about 1 hour to make, and you should start to feel sleepy within 1 hour after drinking it. One warning: Valerian has a bad odor and doesn't taste too pleasant—but it works. (If you can't handle valerian in tea, take it in capsule form and make the tea without it, using 2 teaspoons of passionflower and 3 teaspoons of skullcap.)

    1 cup water
    3 teaspoons dried powdered valerian
    2 teaspoons dried passionflower
    1 teaspoon dried skullcap
       Honey (to taste)

Boil the water. Put the valerian, passionflower, and skullcap in a cup. Pour the water over the herbs. Cover it and steep it for 1 hour. Strain the tea and add honey to taste.

ounces of dried chamomile, ½ ounce of dried St. John's wort, ½ ounce of dried skullcap, and ½ ounce of dried passionflower. This recipe makes about 60 cups of tea. Boil 4 to 6 cups of water in a pot. After the water boils, add 1 tablespoon of the herb mixture for every 2 cups of water.

Take the pot off the heat source and place a lid on it. Let it steep for 10 minutes. Then strain out the herbs and enjoy.

Steep your feet. If you put a lot of stress on yourself, and especially your feet, take the pressure off both by making an herbal footbath. Gould teaches how to make herbal footbaths in her classes and says it is always a student favorite. "Footbaths work on so many levels. The scent, the colors, the heat," she says.

Good herbs for a relaxing footbath are dried roses (the leaves and petals), dried chamomile, and dried lavender. Boil 1 to 2 gallons of water in a pot. Add 2 cups of the herb mixture for each gallon of water. Cover it and let it cool. When it reaches a comfortable temperature—usually as hot as you can stand it—pour it into a small tub big enough for your feet.

Don't worry about straining the water; the pretty colors floating around your ankles add to the relaxing experience.

Soak in your tea. If it makes a good relaxing tea, it also makes a good relaxing bath. You can make a relaxing tea from lemon balm, passionflower, and chamomile, notes Leslie J. Peterson, N.D., a naturopathic physician in Orem, Utah. Combine ½ ounce each of the three dried herbs. Use 1 teaspoon of the mixture for each cup of tea. Try the same combination of herbs in the tub for a soothing herbal bath blend. Make a gallon or so of the tea and pour it into your bath, she says. Then soak your cares of the day away.

Relax in a sea of salts. Toss in some homemade bath salts during your next long, hot bath, advises Gould. Take a cup of sea salt, which you can buy at a health food store, and place it in a glass jar. Add 10 drops of lavender essential oil and 10 drops of chamomile essential oil. Grab about ½ cup of the bath salts and add them to your bathwater.

"I enjoy using bath salts because they are calming and healing," Gould says.

Note: Some essential oils, including those mentioned in this chapter, may cause skin irritation or an allergic reaction in certain individuals. People with sensitive skin should do a patch test before using essential oils.

Luxuriate in serenity bath oil. Ulrich created a "serenity bath oil" recipe that she says helps melt away stress and tension. Pour 2 ounces of almond or grapeseed oil into a jar or bottle. Add 10 drops of lavender essential oil, 10 drops of orange essential oil, and 2 or 3 drops of cedarwood essential oil. Shake well. Add 1 to 2 teaspoons of the bath oil to a full tub of water.

Mix an herbal cocktail. The herb damiana has a reputation as an aphrodisiac, but it also has the ability to quell anxiety, Gould says. To sit back and really relax with damiana, stir yourself up a sweet damiana elixir. Take a jar or bottle and fill it up halfway with dried damiana herb. Fill the rest of the bottle up with an alcoholic beverage of your choice, such as apricot brandy, peach schnapps, or banana liqueur. Shake it a couple of times a day for 2 weeks. Leave it on your counter, out of direct sunlight, during this period so you'll remember to shake it. Then strain the herb out of the liquid. Add a little bit of honey to sweeten the drink, and mix it well. Finally, pour some of the elixir into a small cordial glass and sip. (Store the remainder away from direct sunlight and excessive heat.) "It is very calming to the central nervous system, and it is a great way to relax," Gould says.

Enjoy herbal pops. Remember taking your sweet time savoring a fruity ice pop as a kid? Why not use an herbal pop as a fun way to unwind at the end of the day? Instead of boiling water, boil apple juice, Gould says. Add 1 to 2 teaspoons of dried chamomile or dried lemon balm per cup of juice. Cover and let the herbs steep for 20 minutes. Strain the herbs from the juice. Pour the juice into an ice cube tray. Cover the tray with plastic wrap and place a toothpick in each cube. Freeze until solid.

Knead away tension. Nothing takes away stress and puts you in a calmer mood better than a massage. Combine massage with some serenity herbs and you double the relaxation. Let someone give you a massage, or treat yourself to a relaxing foot or hand massage with herb-infused oils.

To create a relaxing massage oil, choose one or more of the following herbs: dried roses, dried lavender, dried chamomile, and dried comfrey. Place 2 ounces of the mixture in a wide-mouth jar. Pour about 1 pint of almond, apricot, or grapeseed oil over the herbs so that there is at least 2 inches of oil above the herbs, says herbalist Rosemary Gladstar, director of the Sage Mountain Herbal Education Center in East Barre, Vermont, and author of *Herbal Healing for Women*. You may wish to add a drop or two of pure essential oil to scent the mixture. Let the jar stand in a warm place, and shake it every day for 2 weeks. Using a kitchen strainer or cheesecloth, strain the oil.

This supply will be enough for quite a few full-body massages since you need to use only a small amount. Any remaining oil can be stored in your refrigerator for several months.

Spray worries away with lavender. Combine the soothing effects of lavender flowers with lavender essential oil in a floral spray. Mix 1 cup of distilled water with 3 cups of white wine. Add ¾ teaspoon of lavender essential oil and 1 tablespoon of dried lavender flowers. Let the mixture steep in a sunny window for 3 days, then put it in a cooler place for 4 days, Ulrich says. Strain out the dried herb and pour the mix into a spray bottle.

Spray your body or a room when you need a moment of

relaxation. Or add a cupful or two to bathwater. Store the solution in a cool spot away from light, such as in a cupboard.

Take it with you. "You can't live your life at 90 miles an hour all day and then expect to take a teaspoon of something at night and be all better," Gould points out. Keep a bottle of a relaxing herbal tincture with a dropper in your purse or briefcase. Try a combination of chamomile and passionflower, for example. Every few hours, take a few dropperfuls of the tincture in water or juice. "Slowly let your body relax throughout the day," she says.

The Energizing Herbs

Most of us know the meaning of fatigue. Our kids and grandkids frazzle us. The office grind turns us into 5:00 P.M. zombies. We hang on by our fingernails, yearning for the weekends. We feel doomed to low energy.

But we're not.

There's something we can do.

If you should ever find yourself doing lunch with a group of herbalists, something will strike you immediately: You're surrounded by perky people. Despite busy, on-the-go lives—moving from one conference to the next, crossing time zones, delivering lectures, keeping up with new findings, creating new formulas—herbalists manage to remain energized and enthusiastic.

And here's the interesting part: Most of them weren't born that way!

Obviously, they're on to something. But it's not wizardry. It's basic knowledge of the human body, plus some common sense and—you guessed it—a few herbs.

Here's what we know: There are three bad guys in the body that rob us of our energy: toxins, infections, and hormonal imbalances. The liver should take care of toxins; the immune system should stamp out infections; and the endocrine system should keep our hormones in balance. And they all do—so long as we keep them healthy and well-cared-for.

How do we do that? To begin with, by making sound lifestyle and dietary choices, such as getting enough sleep, exercising regularly, and eating plenty of fresh fruits, vegetables, and whole-grain products.

Once these fundamental healthy behaviors are in place, herbal healers say you can use herbs to put more spring in your step and keep your energy high all day. They can help to fortify your liver, bolster your immune system, and keep your hormones in balance.

"We encourage people to take a holistic approach to improving their health," says Mindy Green, a founding and professional member of the American Herbalists Guild, director of educational services for the Herb Research Foundation in Boulder, Colorado, and coauthor of *Aromatherapy: A Complete Guide to the Healing Art.* "Herbal remedies restore energy best when people discontinue abusive behaviors like drinking coffee and smoking cigarettes."

Here are some ways that herbalists keep themselves going strong.

Swap coffee for green tea. If you need a morning wake-up, try green tea. It contains caffeine, but it also has beneficial compounds you won't find in coffee.

"Green tea gives you energy and added benefits, such as antioxidants, that round up free radicals in your cells," says Green, a regular green tea drinker. "I advise steeping the green tea for no more than 3 minutes, or it will taste bitter. Adding a bit of honey to sweeten it is fine."

If you're in a hurry, keep a supply of organic green tea bags on hand. Or infuse 1 teaspoon of organic dried green tea leaves in a cup of boiling water for a few minutes, then strain out the leaves and sip.

Bounce back from sleepless nights. If you find yourself dragging through your morning because you tossed and turned all of the previous night, Green suggests trying a traditional Chinese medicine called schisandra. This herb has been used for centuries for insomnia and physical exhaustion. You can find it in health food stores or order it through the mail.

For tea drinkers, use 1 teaspoon of crushed powder per cup of boiling water. Steep for 10 to 20 minutes, then strain and sip. Drink up to three cups a day to revive your energy.

If you'd rather take schisandra in capsules, the recommended daily amount is 1,500 to 6,000 milligrams split in two doses.

Restore energy with dandelion. That common nuisance of a weed blooming in the cracks of your sidewalk can be a real pal in helping you get the poisons out of your system. "The dandelion root is considered one of the supreme herbs for the liver," says herbalist Rosemary Gladstar, director of the Sage Mountain Herbal Education Center in East Barre, Vermont, and author of *Herbal Healing for Women*.

Loaded with vitamins and minerals, both its root and leaves can help your liver to do a better job of ridding toxins from your body.

Gladstar enjoys sipping dandelion tea or eating a salad abundant with fresh dandelion leaves on a daily basis.

Send fatigue fleeing with an uplifting tea. When your on-the-go lifestyle finds you skipping meals or ordering too many dinners at the drive-thru, your body craves recharging. Try reducing or eliminating feelings of fatigue with this tea prepared by Gladstar.

Collect two parts of raspberry leaf, two parts of nettle

leaf, four parts of peppermint, one part of alfalfa, and one-quarter part of grated gingerroot. Scoop 4 to 6 tablespoons of this herbal blend into a quart of cold water in a saucepan. Bring the tea to a simmer over low heat with the pan covered. Remove the pan from the stove and allow the tea to stand for 20 minutes. Strain out the herbs and drink up to four cups a day.

Gain energy with ginseng. If you're seeking an herb that can go the distance in helping your body overcome stress and fatigue, consider Siberian ginseng. It's especially good as a rejuvenator for women going through menopause because it steps in as a hormonal leveler and mood enhancer, says Gladstar.

Although there are many ways to take ginseng, Gladstar enjoys making a tonic using fresh Siberian ginseng root. Cut a 4-inch ginseng root into slices. Place them in a glass jar with 4 cups of water and seal with a lid. Place the jar in a large pot with enough water to cover about three-fourths of the jar. Cover the pot with a lid; simmer slowly for about 6 hours. Add water if the level gets below one-half. This method provides you with a concentrated ginseng tonic that will help end your energy drain. You need take it only once or twice a month.

For best results, drink a cup of this ginseng tonic at night with a light meal of grains and steamed vegetables. If needed, you can drink another cup in the morning, says Gladstar.

Dine on stimulating soup. When a cold or flu zaps you of your energy and taxes your immune system, consider this herbal soup created by Jennifer Reid, N.D., a naturopathic physician in Gresham, Oregon.

In a vegetable broth base, combine two handfuls of fresh parsley, one large shiitake mushroom (sliced), three slices of fresh ginger, three garlic cloves, and ¼ teaspoon of ground red pepper. You can also add sliced carrots or other favorite soup vegetables. Simmer in a covered pot for 10 minutes. Have up to three cups a day to fend off energy-draining colds and flu.

Ground red pepper (also known as cayenne) can irritate your gastrointestinal tract if you take it on an empty stomach.

This nutrient-rich and calorie-low soup is hot and spicy, says Dr. Reid. The garlic and mushroom fight bacterial and viral invaders; ginger and red pepper aid digestion; and parsley is high in iron and vitamin C.

Keep pace with a stamina formula. If you enjoy working out at the gym, taking brisk walks, or spending hours in the garden, you may want to try the following stamina formula, created by herbalist Kathi Keville, director of the American Herb Association and author of *Herbs for Health and Healing.*

Combine 1 teaspoon of Siberian ginseng root tincture with ½ teaspoon each of tinctures of schisandra berries, ginseng root (American or Korean), saw palmetto berries, and licorice root. Take half a dropperful twice a day or as needed to boost your stamina.

Ginseng and schisandra seem to help improve endurance, muscle strength, cardiovascular fitness, and mental clarity. Licorice appears to increase energy storage in your muscles, while saw palmetto may aid in building muscles.

Smart Healing
with Herbs

Columbus discovered America by accident. He wasn't after real estate. He was after herbs.

Queen Isabella . . . trade route to India . . . herbs and spices. Every American schoolchild knows the story. But exactly what made these herbs so desirable that men would risk their lives plying the briny deeps to get them? The same thing that makes modern medicines so valuable: their curative powers.

Today we can get even the rarest herbs through the mail or at the health food store down the street. But availability isn't enough. Knowing how to use them is just as important.

If you are socked with a nagging headache but are reluctant to reach for ibuprofen, what else can you take? If you feel a cold coming on but dread the drowsiness delivered by over-the-counter capsules, is there a better alternative? If you need an energy boost but know that coffee isn't a healthy choice, what is healthier and works as well?

Try taming that throbbing head with white willow. Calm the cold with echinacea. Fend off fatigue with a whiff of peppermint.

When herbs are used as a remedy, one basic rule always applies: Although usually quite safe, they still must be treated with the same caution that is applied to prescription and over-the-counter medications. Beyond that, care must be taken in choosing the right herb in the right form and in the right dose. For instance, ginkgo makes a great-tasting tea, but if you're looking to sharpen your memory, a standardized extract capsule is the best medicinal choice, says Mindy Green, a founding and professional member of the American Herbalists Guild, director of educational services for the Herb Research Foundation in Boulder, Colorado, and coauthor of *Aromatherapy: A Complete Guide to the Healing Art.*

"At times, herbs can be used instead of a drug that has harmful side effects," says Jennifer Reid, N.D., a naturopathic physician in Gresham, Oregon. Sometimes herbs can complement prescription medication. Whichever way they are used, it's best if the choice of herb or herbs is formulated to fit the specific needs of the individual.

Check with your doctor before taking herbs in place of your prescription medications, especially those for chronic conditions such as diabetes or high blood pressure. Also, get your physician's stamp of approval before you add herbs to your medications in the hope of achieving better results. If you're taking a digitalis-type medication for your heart condition, for example, you could develop serious problems by adding hawthorn.

Most people don't develop side effects from taking herbs. But if you suddenly develop skin rashes, forehead-tapping headaches, mild diarrhea, or nausea lasting longer than 2 days, your body might be telling you that it doesn't want these substances. Work with a health care practitioner qualified in the use of herbal remedies to determine if these symptoms mean you need to reduce the amount of herb, change the specific formula, or switch to a different formula altogether.

Two special cautions: Women should stop using herbs as soon as they know they are pregnant. And everyone needs to practice extra caution when using essential oils—extracts distilled from the roots, resins, bark, wood, fruit, leaves, and flowers of plants. Potent and complex, essential oils should *never* be swallowed because ingesting even a few drops can be toxic. They are best used externally in diluted forms. The few exceptions are noted at the end of this book.

The herbal remedies offered by qualified professionals for the health conditions that follow are readily available at health food stores, from mail-order catalogs, and, in some cases, even at the supermarket or drugstore. They were selected because they are easy to use or simple to make. More important, top herbalists and alternative medicine experts regard them as safe with few, if any, side effects.

Acne

Acne isn't just kid stuff. Skin problems can continue or make a comeback in your thirties, forties, and fifties. Why? Too much sebum, an oily substance secreted by glands in your skin. Sebum collects dirt and bacteria, clogging pores. Hormonal fluctuations, stress, fatty diets, and even the harsh ingredients in some cosmetics can shift sebum production into high gear.

The result? A variety of blemish types. If a tiny hair follicle becomes plugged, you get a whitehead. When this plug rises to the skin's surface and meets the air, it darkens and becomes a blackhead. Should the blockage become inflamed or infected, or if it ruptures, you get the frustrating, sometimes painful eruptions known as cystic acne.

Herbalists recommend attacking acne in two ways. First, control it from the inside out with herbs that may help your body eliminate waste material more effectively and bring your hormones to normal levels. Second, use gentle but effective herbal cleansers and moisturizers. Try these techniques recommended by herbal experts.

For cleansing, take root. Burdock root has a long tradition of use for skin problems. Herbalists believe it works by helping the liver eliminate waste more effectively. Take one capsule of dried burdock or 30 drops of burdock root tincture with meals three times a day. Or make a batch of strong burdock tea. Use 1 teaspoon of dried, chopped burdock root per cup of boiling water. Steep for 10 to 20 minutes, then strain and sip. Steeping overnight makes an even stronger brew. Have a cup or two daily to fight acne.

Increase bile flow with dandelion. Dandelion has a reputation as a cleansing herb. It contains bitter compounds that can increase bile flow and stimulate the liver. The benefit? Your body eliminates waste more efficiently, which leads to clearer skin. Some herbalists suggest you take a teaspoon of dandelion tincture daily, diluted in 8 ounces of water. Sip throughout the day.

Cleanse with oatmeal. Make a daily habit of removing dirt and excess oil from your face—gently. Wash your face with an unscented oatmeal soap. Or prepare a simple oatmeal scrub by grinding rolled oats in a food processor, clean coffee grinder, or blender. Mix 2 teaspoons of the oats with about 1 tablespoon of water to form a paste. Gently wash your face with the mixture, then rinse with warm or lukewarm water. Oatmeal removes dirt and oil without stripping all the natural oils from your skin.

• *Herb at a Glance* •

Aloe. Good for minor skin rashes, scrapes, cuts, and burns

Fight bacteria with lavender essential oil. Restore a clear complexion by placing one or two drops of pure essential oil of lavender directly on your blemish as needed. Unlike most essential oils, lavender can be applied directly to the skin in small amounts, without having to be diluted in a carrier oil. Lavender oil is great for a variety of skin conditions because it attacks bacteria and eases pain and swelling.

Moisturize to prevent breakouts. A light moisturizer actually helps acne-prone skin. Mix a drop or two of lavender essential oil with an ounce of light oil such as jojoba or sunflower and apply at night. Why add oil to skin that's already breaking out? Herbal beauty experts say that moisturized skin is less likely to overproduce oil and be at risk for acne.

Age Spots

Age spots may have more to do with overexposure to the sun than the accumulation of birthdays. These dark brown blotches—also called liver spots—are the result of years of sun exposure.

When the prime targets—the face, neck, chest, forearms, and hands—are bombarded by the sun's ultraviolet light year after year, the skin responds by producing melanin, a naturally dark pigment. At first, age spots usually look just like freckles or small moles. Over time, though, they can darken, grow, and multiply, especially if you keep exposing them to the sun.

Dermatologists advise wearing sunscreen and avoiding the sun to reduce the occurrence of new age spots and the continued growth of existing spots. Herbal beauty experts suggest going two steps further: First, use herbal treatments that safely fade and peel away the upper layer of overpigmented, blotchy skin. Then, apply moisturizing formulas that promote the growth of new skin cells, which can make skin look fresher.

Peel sun damage away with elderflowers. In combination, lemon juice and fresh or dried elderflowers help bleach and remove age spots over time. Both contain alpha hydroxy acids that stimulate peeling of the skin's upper layer. Age spots fade and, over time, slough away as natural acids remove old, dead cells and surface discoloration.

Combine 1 tablespoon of fresh or dried elderflowers and 1 teaspoon of lemon juice in a mini food processor or blender. Add just enough water to form a paste. Apply with your fingers to the age spots, being careful to avoid your eyes and lips. It may sting a bit. Leave the paste on for no more than 5 minutes, then rinse it off with lukewarm water. Apply three times per week. Expect to see age spots fade within 3 months.

Peel with parsley. You can also create an effective face peel using lemon juice, a little water, and chopped parsley in place of elderflowers. Follow the directions above for making and using this all-natural peel.

Allergies

Allergies are abnormal reactions to everyday substances like dust mites, pet dander, and mold spores. When your immune system misidentifies these harmless substances as dangerous invaders, your body goes overboard in releasing invasion-fighting chemicals, including histamine. Histamine produces the symptoms of an allergic reaction: sniffles, skin inflammation, indigestion, and headache. In rare cases, usually involving food, drug, or insect allergies, it can even cause a life-threatening body-wide reaction, including breathing difficulties and a dangerous plunge in blood pressure.

• Herb at a Glance •

Basil. Good for diarrhea without any other symptoms and for fever associated with colds and flu

---

Standard medical care for most allergies calls for decongestants, antihistamines, and, sometimes, allergy shots. The decongestants open clogged nasal passages. Antihistamines block the effect of histamine. And allergy shots slowly expose your body to substances it reacts to so that you gradually become desensitized.

Although these medications are effective, some of them can cause drowsiness and insomnia and, in some people, raised blood pressure. Herbalists and alternative medical experts suggest using the following safe plant remedies instead. If you find that your symptoms of sneezing, wheezing, or coughing aren't reduced by these remedies or over-the-counter medicines you've tried, it might be time to visit your doctor.

Dry out watery eyes with eyebright. If allergies leave you with weepy, watery eyes, turn to eyebright. Herbalists say that this herb naturally tones and strengthens the ocular membranes behind the eyes and can stop eyewatering. Take 1 to 4 milligrams of eyebright as a tincture three times a day, as needed.

Breathe easy with ginkgo. The ginkgo tree, often planted in Japanese temple gardens, has an ancient reputation for bolstering the kidneys, lungs, and digestive system and for restoring vitality. Used by some natural healers specifically for allergies, ginkgo contains compounds called ginkgolides that may counter spasms of the bronchial muscles when your immune system is exposed to an allergen like pollen or animal dander. As a result, you can breathe comfortably instead of wheezing. Take 20 to 30 drops of ginkgo tincture up to four times a day. You can dilute the dose in water, juice, or herbal tea.

Season with garlic. Garlic contains high concentrations of the compound quercetin, noted for reducing the severity of inflammatory reactions. If you have allergies, add generous amounts of garlic to your meals.

Altitude Sickness

"Breathtaking" may describe panoramic views from pristine mountaintops—but fast climbs, mountain drives, or even ski-lift rides can also take your breath away.

Altitude sickness is related directly to elevation. At sea level, oxygen molecules in your blood are dense and rich. But at 16,000 feet above sea level, your blood contains one-third less oxygen. When your body is deprived of adequate oxygen, your brain, heart, lungs, and nervous system are affected. Without proper precautions, you may develop dizziness, breathlessness, fatigue, headaches, nausea, and even vomiting. The higher and faster you climb, the worse the symptoms may become.

Fortunately, you can minimize, or even avoid, altitude sickness by working in harmony with Mother Nature's medicinal garden.

Stave off stress with Siberian ginseng. Walking, skiing, or simply vacationing in high-altitude terrain can be quite an adjustment, especially if you normally reside at low altitudes. Start preparing your body a few days before any cloud-climbing expedition by taking Siberian ginseng capsules. This herb bolsters your body's resistance to stress, especially environmental stress. Check the bottle's label for dosage information.

Sip a spicy garlic soup. Spoon up this herbal soup to forestall altitude-related discomfort. Simply combine generous amounts of fresh garlic, dill, fennel, tomatoes, onions, hot peppers, canned soybeans (they cook faster than dried), celery, carrots, and parsley in a few cups of water and simmer for 20 minutes. Garlic is the key, but all these ingredients work together to help keep your blood from thickening as you gain altitude.

Keep a clear head with ginkgo. Increase your chances for a trip free of headaches and dizziness by taking 120 milligrams of standardized ginkgo extract daily for several days beforehand. Studies have demonstrated that ginkgo leaves make blood vessels in the brain more flexible, allowing for better circulation. Ginkgo also thins the blood, helping reduce headaches and dizziness by supplying more oxygen to the brain.

Anemia

If you have anemia, you may feel weary and weak. The simplest activities become energy sapping. Anemia is the medical term for a reduction in red blood cell count. Red blood cells contain hemoglobin, a protein that transports oxygen to muscles, body tissues, and organs—where it fortifies and energizes. Without sufficient red blood cells, your body won't receive enough oxygen to function optimally, leaving you feeling tired, cold, lousy, and lifeless.

How do you know if you're anemic? A simple blood test is the best indicator.

Conventional doctors often prescribe iron supplements in the form of ferrous sulfate to treat iron deficiency anemia, the most common type of anemia. Some herbal experts, however, say these supplements may not be fully absorbed by the body and can cause constipation and stomach distress. Taking these supplements for prolonged periods, say some herbalists, may spark the formation of free radicals, oxygen-stealing molecules that contribute to such diseases as colon cancer and heart disease.

Instead of taking iron supplements, bolster your diet with dark green leafy vegetables and foods that are naturally rich in iron, such as roasted dark turkey meat or steamed clams. Then supplement those smart food choices with some of these herbal remedies.

Boost iron with yellow dock root. This bitter-tasting herb is believed by some herbalists to be the best herbal antidote for iron deficiency. Try commercially made yellow dock capsules, following label directions. Many people find that their iron levels return to normal within a few weeks to a month.

Brew an iron-rich tea. Fortify your body's iron supply by drinking two cups of this "iron tea" each day. Mix 2 teaspoons of yellow dock root with ½ teaspoon each of nettle leaves, dandelion root, beet root, and licorice root. Boil this herbal blend in 3 cups of water. Then turn down the heat and simmer the mixture for 5 minutes. Turn off the heat and let it steep for another 20 minutes. Strain out the herbs before drinking the tea.

Munch a dandelion-dressed salad. Fresh dandelion leaves contain iron as well as magnesium, which assists your body in using iron more efficiently. Make a tasty salad dressing by cutting several handfuls of dandelion leaves (use only leaves from a pesticide-free yard). Rinse them to make sure they're free of dirt, and toss them into a blender. Add oil, vinegar, and herbs and spices of your choice. Blend until the mixture is pureed. Then pour over a salad loaded with kale, spinach, parsley, and other dark leafy greens.

Anxiety

Anxiety is the dread of the not-yet-known. It's that churning sensation in the pit of your stomach when the phone rings unexpectedly at 4:00 A.M., that mounting tension when the plumber mutters his third "Hmmmm" while examining your kitchen sink.

• Herb at a Glance •

Bearberry. Good for chronic bladder problems, including urinary tract infections

---

Lingering anxiety blocks concentration and ignites irritability and sleepless nights—as well as chip-and-dip feeding frenzies. Unchecked, anxiety can elevate your blood pressure and heart rate and make you more susceptible to serious conditions, such as heart disease.

If the anxiety you're feeling is so overwhelming that you are severely distressed, it's a good idea to check with a medical doctor or professional psychotherapist.

You can begin controlling mild or moderate anxiety, however, with calm breathing. When you're anxious, you may breathe shallowly or even hold your breath. By contrast, slow, deep breathing calms your nervous system. So take a deep breath—then rely on these herbal helpers to help you ditch the jitters.

Restore calm with valerian. Soothe an overly excited nervous system by taking one or two capsules (100 to 300 milligrams each) of valerian or 30 to 60 drops of valerian tincture three times a day. Doctors of alternative medicine routinely prescribe valerian in place of diazepam (Valium), alprazolam (Xanax), or other prescription drugs for mild and moderate cases of anxiety.

Rely on kava kava. To subdue feelings of fear and anger, try kava kava, a tropical plant that thrives in the humid South Pacific. Kava kava contains kavalactones, a group of resinous compounds that relax mind and body. Take one capsule (100 milligrams) or 30 drops of standardized kava root tincture three times a day during anxious times. Studies have shown that kava acts on the limbic system, the emotional control center of the brain, subduing feelings of fear and anger while enhancing feelings of pleasure.

Sniff out anxiety with angelica essential oil. Prevent uneasy feelings from mushrooming into a panic attack by keeping handy a bottle of angelica essential oil. The essential oil extracted from this herb restores calm and composure. Put a drop of angelica oil on a hankie and sniff its healing aroma whenever you feel your anxiety escalating.

Arthritis

If you picture a hunched-over, knobby-jointed grandmother when you think of arthritis, take another look. Arthritis pain knows no age limits. More than 100 types can affect people at all stages of life.

Two of the most common forms, osteoarthritis and rheumatoid arthritis, don't usually hit until we're in our forties. Osteoarthritis, the wear-and-tear type, erodes the soft, spongy cartilage that cushions joints, leading to joint pain and stiffness. Rheumatoid arthritis, on the other hand, is an autoimmune disease that prompts the body's own immune system to turn on itself. It causes the membrane that lubricates each joint to swell. Other symptoms of rheumatoid arthritis include redness in the joints, fever, fatigue, and loss of appetite.

Having arthritis does not necessarily mean enduring a lifetime of pain. Eating healthfully and making other lifestyle changes can soften the symptoms. Certain herbs can also improve mobility and reduce pain and stiffness.

Rub down with lemon and sandalwood. An herbal rub made with essential oils can ease joint pain and inflammation. Make your own by starting with a small jar of petroleum jelly. Scoop out a tablespoon of the jelly. Then add 20 drops of essential oil of lemon and 20 drops of essential oil of sandalwood to the jar. Mix the oil well into the petroleum jelly. Rub this mixture on sore joints four times a day.

Improve joint mobility with ginger. Ginger's anti-inflammatory qualities may help curb the pain, swelling, and morning stiffness often associated with rheumatoid arthritis. Slice a piece of fresh ginger. Put a few slivers into a tea ball. Place the tea ball in a cup, pour freshly boiled water over it, and steep for 10 minutes. Make sure the tea has cooled to a comfortable temperature before sipping.

Stimulate the liver and kidneys with two roots. Herbalists believe that arthritis may improve when the body eliminates wastes more efficiently. To achieve this, they turn to dandelion and burdock, which encourage a healthy liver and kidneys. Try this anti-arthritis tea: Boil 1 teaspoon of dried dandelion root and 1 teaspoon of dried burdock root in 3 cups of water for 5 minutes. Strain and sip throughout the day. If the taste is too bitter for your liking, add a bit of honey.

Suppress the pain with hot pepper. Apply ground red pepper in cream form to achy joints to make pain disappear. Hot pepper (cayenne) contains two important ache-fighting chemicals: capsaicin and salicylates. Capsaicin relieves pain by unleashing endorphins, your body's homemade feel-good chemicals. Salicylates have aspirin-like properties. Apply capsaicin cream directly to painful arthritic joints four times daily. Always thoroughly wash your hands afterward to avoid getting the cream in your eyes.

Asthma

Classic asthma-attack triggers include exposure to air pollutants, pet dander, pollen, or mold. A bad cold, exercise, stress, crying, anger, or even hearty laughter can also bring on symptoms. Further, hormone fluctuations during menstruation or pregnancy may cause heightened asthma symptoms for some sensitive women.

No matter what the cause of your asthma, the scenario

inside your lungs is the same: During an attack, the tubes that allow oxygen to pass into your lungs tighten and swell. At the same time, these passages produce a lot of mucus, which further clogs airways. Breathing becomes difficult, and you may wheeze, cough, or feel tightness in your chest.

Asthma should never be ignored: It's important to see your doctor for a treatment plan. He's likely to prescribe drugs that will quickly relax constricted breathing passages and reduce inflammation. You should never stop taking your asthma medication without your doctor's approval. That said, you may be able to reduce your dependence on these medications and breathe easier with the following herbal treatments.

Go for ginkgo. For centuries, Asian healers have relied on extracts of ginkgo leaves to safely treat asthmatic conditions. The beauty of ginkgo is that it interferes with a protein in the blood responsible for causing spasms in bronchial tubes. For best results, take 60 to 240 milligrams of standardized ginkgo extract a day. If you exceed that amount, you risk diarrhea, irritability, and restlessness.

Shrink symptoms with evening primrose. Evening primrose oil may reduce the airway inflammation associated with asthma. Experts recommend two 500-milligram capsules of evening primrose oil three times a day.

Let coleus forskohlii relax bronchial muscles. Coleus forskohlii has been shown in studies to be as effective as prescription asthma drugs, without causing the shakiness, tremors, and other unwanted side effects associated with those medications. Keep asthma under control by swallowing 50 milligrams two or three times a day. Look for standardized extracts of this herb that contain 18 percent forskolin, the substance experts believe is the active ingredient in this herb.

Tone down swelling with licorice. To reduce inflammation, select a standardized licorice-root product (such as capsules) that contains 12 percent glycyrrhizin. Take two capsules three times daily.

Athlete's Foot

Just because it's called athlete's foot doesn't mean you can get itchy, peeling, cracked feet only in the gym. You can pick up your own case by walking barefoot around swimming pools, locker rooms, even your own bathroom—if someone else with the infection has been there before you.

Athlete's foot occurs when a fungus sets up house in the damp skin between your toes and on the bottom and sides of your feet. There, it quickly goes to work, causing all kinds of mischief to the skin of your feet. Ditch the itch and soothe your toes with herbal remedies that some natural healers say not only help to oust the fungal infection but also make you less susceptible to future invasions.

Mix an antifungal soak. Tea tree essential oil helps fight athlete's foot fungus. Put it to work in a footbath: Once a day, mix five to seven drops of tea tree oil into 4 ounces of warm water in a tub big enough to hold your feet. If you need more liquid to cover the affected area, you can double this recipe. Soak your feet for 20 minutes to ease the itching and soothe cracked skin and infected nails. Then dry your feet thoroughly with a clean towel and put on clean cotton socks.

Follow up with a calendula salve. After you've used an antifungal soak for 3 days, add calendula cream or salve to your routine. The petals of this yellow and orange flower have been used in traditional skin-healing remedies. Look for calendula cream or salve in a health food store or through mail order. Apply after soaking and drying your feet. You can use the calendula salve up to three times a day.

Control the itch all day with ginger—and more. Fight the itch of athlete's foot with a light, fragrant foot powder made with ginger and tea tree oil. Both herbs have antiseptic and antifungal properties, so they fight the fungus and can help control bacterial infections in skin already inflamed by athlete's foot.

Combine ½ cup of powdered arrowroot, ½ cup of cosmetic clay, and 2 tablespoons of powdered ginger; cover the mixture and shake it. Add 20 drops of tea tree essential oil and shake again. Store in a covered, dark glass jar in a cool, dry place. Apply as needed to your feet. This powder also helps control moisture, making your feet a less hospitable place for the athlete's foot fungus to breed.

Bad Breath

The culprit behind offensive mouth fumes may be a nighttime's worth of germs that multiply gleefully before you can brush and gargle in the morning. Aromatic food and drink, such as garlic-laden pasta, raw onions, or coffee, may also leave a lingering scent that contributes to bad breath. If chronic bad breath hounds you for weeks, see your doctor or dentist to check for serious health conditions such as diabetes, liver or kidney problems, a bad tooth, or infected gums.

Of course, regular brushing and flossing are the first steps to take against garden-variety halitosis. Add to this daily dental routine the following herbal mouth fresheners for naturally sweet breath.

Munch some parsley. To quell common food-related mouth odor, chew parsley after meals. This

> • *Herb at a Glance* •
> **Burdock.** Good for psoriasis, eczema, and acne

green sprig contains chlorophyll, a well-known breath deodorizer. Or skip the sprigs and swallow parsley capsules such as BreathAsure (containing parsley and sunflower oil).

Crunch cardamom. This popular Arabian spice is full of cineole, a powerful antiseptic that kills bad-breath bacteria. You can buy whole cardamom pods at health food stores and some supermarkets. Rejuvenate your breath by splitting the pods and chewing on a few of the seeds found inside. Discreetly spit out the seeds when you're finished.

Concoct a spicy mouthwash. Homemade cinnamon mouthwash curbs unpleasant mouth odor as well as or better than some brand-name mouth rinses. Combine 10½ tablespoons of ground cinnamon with 1¼ cups of apple-cider vinegar in a bottle with a tight-fitting lid. Let stand for 2 weeks, shaking twice daily (morning and night). Then strain this solution through cheesecloth or a coffee filter and store it in a clean glass or plastic bottle. To use it, swish and gargle for 1 minute to fight bad breath.

Try a minty anti-halitosis tea. Kill the germs that cause bad breath with peppermint tea. Drink a cup whenever your breath needs freshening. The aromatic oil in this mint acts as a potent antiseptic.

Bites and Stings

When mosquitoes bite or bees sting, their attacks can cause redness, fire-hot pain, unrelenting itching, swelling, and, sometimes, skin infection.

The annoying winged creatures fall into two categories: bloodsuckers and stingers. Mosquitoes, fleas, black flies, deer flies, and itsy-bitsy mites want to suck your

Get the Sting Out

If you get bitten or stung by an insect, you can quickly ease the pain and swelling by using widely available plantain or chickweed plants, says Angela Stengler, N.D., a naturopathic physician and herbal author in Oceanside, California.

Plantain grows wild along roadsides and may even be in your own backyard. Look for a low-to-the-ground plant with egg-shaped, smooth leaves that are 3 to 8 inches long. The small white flowers grow elongated spikes, which protrude from the middle of the plant. Plantain grows from March until October.

Chickweed often grows under trees (especially oaks) and in other shady places. Its tiny star-shaped white flowers grow on a tangled stem along with pairs of small, succulent light-green leaves.

To use, pick a handful of fresh plantain or chickweed leaves. Make certain there is no dirt on the leaves. Also make sure there are no neighboring poison ivy plants that may have spread their oils to the healing plants.

Rub the leaves together in your hands until they are juicy. Place the wet leaves on the bite or sting for 15 to 30 minutes. If a gauze pad is available, place it over the wet leaves and fasten it with a larger piece of rolled gauze.

blood. Bees, wasps, yellow jackets, and velvet ants defend themselves by jabbing you with the tiny, poisoned harpoons in their butts. (Of these, only the honeybee leaves her stinger behind in your skin, along with a sac of venom.) If you're stung by a bee, first safely remove the stinger and sac by scraping them away with your thumbnail or a credit card.

Note: People allergic to insect venom can develop life-threatening reactions. If you have difficulty breathing or develop hives on your arms, legs, or torso, call your local emergency medical number, or head to the nearest hospital, pronto.

Otherwise, try these simple herbal soothers for fast relief from the pain, itch, infection, and swelling.

Stop pain and itching with peppermint. Get fast, long-lasting relief by rubbing a tiny droplet of peppermint essential oil into the bull's-eye center of bites and stings. Peppermint essential oil has been used traditionally as an antiseptic and local anesthetic. It cools the area, reducing itching and pain. Thoroughly wash your hands after application so that you won't irritate your eyes.

Dab on calendula. This herb encourages tissue healing and acts as a natural, infection-fighting antiseptic. Make a calendula tea, using about 1 tablespoon of the dried herb per cup of boiling water. Let it steep for 5 minutes, then strain and let it cool. Dip a cotton ball into the calendula tea and dab it on bites or stings four or five times daily until the skin has healed.

Soothe inflammation with echinacea. For stubborn bug bites that stay swollen, ease the inflammation with an echinacea poultice. For a small bite, combine 1 teaspoon of echinacea tincture and 1 teaspoon of water with enough bentonite clay to create a thick paste. The clay can be purchased in some health food stores or herb specialty shops. (You can double this recipe for larger or multiple bites.) Dab the mixture on the bite and cover it with an adhesive strip bandage. Reapply the paste and change the dressing twice a day.

A large German study demonstrated that echinacea, when used topically, regenerates tissue, reduces swelling, and spurs the body's immune system into action.

As an alternative, drink 60 drops of echinacea tincture mixed in ¼ cup of warm water three times a day for up to 2 weeks.

Breastfeeding

As natural as breastfeeding is, sometimes nature needs a little nudge. You want to make sure your breasts have enough milk for your newborn—not too little or too much. And being a good mom means being good to yourself as well as your baby. You may need relief from sore, cracked, or even bleeding nipples after nursing.

If you think your milk production could use a boost, discuss with your doctor the gentle, safe herbal remedies mentioned below. While taking any medication—natural or otherwise—is usually prohibited during breastfeeding, some herbalists recommend a class of botanicals known as galactagogues for nursing mothers. These herbs have been recognized as milk enhancers for hundreds, if not thousands, of years.

Build your milk supply with herbal tea. Daily stress can prevent you from producing enough milk to satisfy your baby. You can restore calmness and help boost your milk production by sipping a multi-herbal blend.

Combine one part each of oatstraw and chamomile and one-half part each of lavender and nettle. Add a pinch of fennel seed for each cup of tea you make. Steep 1 teaspoon of this blend in a cup of boiled water for 15 minutes, then strain and sip. Research suggests that lavender, chamomile, and oatstraw are calming agents, while nettle and fennel promote lactation.

Try a simple fennel brew. Pungent fennel seed displays mild estrogen-like properties, and for centuries, women have used it to promote milk production. Try it yourself with a tasty fennel tea. Use 2 teaspoons of crushed seeds per cup of boiling water, steep it for at least 5 minutes, strain, and sip. Have up to three cups each day.

Soothe sore nipples with aloe. Heal the nipple area and ease pain with aloe vera gel. Snip a leaf from an aloe plant, slit it open lengthwise, and scrape out the cool, clear gel. Spread it on your nipples. It's best to use the gel after breastfeeding—and be sure to wash it off thoroughly before your next feeding. Aloe's bitterness is not something a baby would enjoy.

Breast Pain

If your breasts feel uncomfortable, swollen, or achy, the hormone estrogen may be to blame. When estrogen levels are high—usually just before and during menstruation—one or both breasts may swell and become achy, tender, and even lumpy. Estrogen stimulates fluid retention in breast tissues.

Levels of discomfort vary. One woman may feel mild tenderness; another, excruciating pain. Doctors say that breast pain is very common and usually not a cause for alarm. Most of the time, your menstrual cycle is the cause.

You can reduce discomfort by cutting back on or eliminating caffeine-rich foods and drinks, including coffee, black teas, colas, and chocolates. All contain substances that may contribute to breast pain. Also, limit your intake of animal fats, which seem to raise estrogen levels. Plan your meals around organic whole grains, vegetables, and fruits, which help to keep your hormone levels in balance.

Now you're ready for step two. Herbalists favor these botanicals to correct hormonal imbalances and assist your body in processing hormones efficiently.

Tame the pain with black cohosh. Studies demonstrate that this pain-relieving herb also acts as a mild sedative and reduces swelling in tender breasts. Take a dropperful of black cohosh tincture (also called an extract) in tea, juice, or warm water three or four times a day for several months until the symptoms dissipate.

Curb the ache with evening primrose. If you've eliminated caffeine from your diet but still experience painful and swollen breasts before your menstrual period arrives, natural healers recommend evening primrose oil, an effective anti-inflammatory herb. Take one or two 500-milligram capsules two or three times a day.

Reduce swelling with an herbal combo. Ease breast tenderness and pain caused by swollen lymph nodes by mixing a simple herbal combination. Combine equal amounts of tinctures of cleavers, milk thistle, rosemary, and sarsaparilla. Drink ¼ to ½ teaspoon of this mix three to five times a day, in water, juice, or tea, until the lumps start to go away. These herbs help to move fluids through your body's lymphatic system and prevent them from pooling in lymph nodes. They also help balance hormone levels.

Bronchitis

Call bronchitis the never-quit cough. That deep, raspy, painful hacking can last for weeks, thanks to upper respiratory infections that inflame and irritate the airways leading to your lungs.

If you have bronchitis, your lungs are probably congested with mucus, creating an ideal breeding ground for infection. It's important to reduce your risk of lung infections, including pneumonia, by getting this mucus up and out. If your cough gets worse or you feel weak, tired, short of

> • *Herb at a Glance* •
> **Calendula.** Good for reducing topical inflammation and fighting infections

breath, or feverish, it is important to go to your doctor to rule out pneumonia. The only way to know for sure is to have a chest x-ray. If you haven't reached that stage yet, follow these herbal strategies to calm a hard-to-shake cough and clear congested lungs.

Inhale eucalyptus vapors. Commission E, a group of scientists that advises the German government about herbal medicine, says that eucalyptus essential oil is an effective expectorant for loosening phlegm. Inhale eucalyptus vapors to treat bronchitis and its persistent cough. One way is to create your own personal steam bath.

Place several cups of water in a tea kettle and bring to a boil. Carefully pour the steaming water into a bowl and add several drops of eucalyptus essential oil. Drape a large towel over your head and lean over the bowl about 12 inches or so, close enough to feel the steam without burning yourself. Breathe deeply, inhaling the eucalyptus vapors as they waft toward your nostrils.

Soothe the mucous membranes with mullein. Relieve inflamed mucous membranes and help remove mucus from the lungs with mullein tea. Steep 2 teaspoons of this dried herb in a cup of just-boiled water for about 10 minutes. Strain and drink. Have up to three cups a day. As a bonus, mullein also reduces swollen glands, which often accompany bronchitis.

Rub in spicy relief. Reduce lung congestion with this easy-to-assemble herbal vapor rub recommended by natural healers. In a glass bottle, combine ¼ teaspoon eucalyptus essential oil, ⅛ teaspoon peppermint essential oil, ⅛ teaspoon thyme essential oil, and ¼ cup olive oil. Shake to mix evenly. Gently massage the mixture onto your chest and throat as needed.

Calm the cough with plantain. English plantain has a worldwide reputation as an effective cough suppressant and bacteria fighter. Make a hot tea, using 1 teaspoon of dried plantain per cup of water. Steep until cool, then drink as needed.

Bruises

Bruises happen when blood vessels break beneath the surface of your skin and leak small amounts of blood, which can cause pain and swelling. You may find you bruise more easily as you get older because collagen—the connective tissue that cushions skin—breaks down, leaving blood vessels more vulnerable to bumps and collisions. Certain medications, including blood thinners like aspirin, also increase your risk of bruising.

Most bruises heal on their own within a few weeks. You can hasten the healing process and ease the pain and unsightliness with these botanical treatments.

Reach for arnica. Also called mountain daisy, arnica contains an active ingredient, helenalin, that clinical studies show relieves pain and reduces swelling from bruises. You can buy arnica creams, gels, and ointments wherever herbal products are sold. Use arnica only on unbroken skin, and stop using it if your skin becomes red, itchy, or inflamed after applying the arnica. Never take arnica internally.

Call on calendula. The ancient Greeks swore by these bright yellow and orange flowers when it came to mending bruises. To craft an herbal poultice, soak 1 tablespoon of dried calendula flowers in an equal amount of warm water until the flowers are rehydrated—they should look more like fresh flowers. (If fresh calendula is available, simply crush some petals.) Then place the petals directly on the bruise, keeping the herb in place for 3 to 4 hours with an adhesive strip. Use gauze and tape for a larger area. The sooner you apply the poultice, the better the chance you'll avert severe swelling, pain, and discoloration.

Chill the black-and-blues with parsley ice cubes. Have this icy herbal remedy on hand in the freezer so that you can put the brakes on swelling quickly next time you're nursing a new bruise. Put a handful of parsley and ¼ cup of water in a blender, then blend until slushy. Fill ice cube trays halfway with this mixture and freeze. When you need relief, wrap a parsley ice cube in gauze or a thin cloth and place it directly on the bruised site for 15 to 20 minutes. Parsley is a traditional bruise mender, and the ice will help relieve or prevent swelling.

Stock up on flower-powered herbal ice. Place 1 teaspoon of chamomile flowers and 1 teaspoon of lavender flowers in a pan. Add 1 cup of boiling water, cover the pan, and let the mixture steep for about 15 minutes. Strain out the herbs. Freeze the tea mixture in an ice cube tray. When the cubes are frozen solid, pop them out and store in a plastic freezer bag. When the next bruise occurs, wrap a thin cloth around an herbal ice cube and apply it to the bruise for 10 to 20 minutes; repeat every 2 hours.

In addition to the inflammation-soothing powers of the ice, the chamomile and lavender in these bruise cubes discourage swelling and promote faster healing.

Burns and Scalds

Although it's hard to imagine a more painful wound, most burns and scalds are minor and can be treated safely at home without the need for a trip to the emergency room. Prepare by stocking up on appropriate herbal remedies. You'll be ready to minimize pain and skin damage—quickly.

Before applying any herbal treatment, immediately run

cool water over the burned area. This cools the skin and relieves pain. Then reach for these herbal soothers and skin healers.

Treat it with aloe. Simply snap off one of the spiky outer leaves of an aloe plant and slit it open lengthwise. Squeeze the transparent gel out of the leaf and onto burned skin.

The clear, cooling gel inside this common, easy-growing plant offers protection against pain, reduces swelling, and dilates capillaries, which brings more blood—and more of the body's own team of skin menders—to burn-damaged skin. Aloe also contains vitamin C, vitamin E, and zinc—nutrients that speed wound healing.

Reduce scarring with two skin-friendly herbs. Calendula and comfrey have earned reputations as skin menders. Researchers believe that triterpenes in calendula spur the growth of new cells and that allantoin in comfrey hastens tissue repair. Apply a salve containing calendula and comfrey to minor burns. Never use comfrey on deep burns or on burns that show signs of infection, like redness, puffiness, or oozing. It can heal surface skin so quickly that it may trap the infection underneath.

Cool the burn with a botanical bath. Fill your tub with cool water, then head for the kitchen and prepare this herbal burn fighter.

Bring 1 quart of water to a boil, then turn the heat off and pour in ¼ cup each of comfrey leaves, plantain leaves, and calendula flowers. Stir in three drops of lavender essential oil and 1 cup of colloidal oatmeal (a finely powdered oatmeal available at drugstores) or regular oatmeal milled in a

> • *Herb at a Glance* •
> **Chamomile.** Good for soothing an irritated stomach and easing muscle spasms

Be Ready for Burns!

Even a small burn can hit you hard in the pain department. Here are important tips from experts to minimize pain and speed healing of first- and second-degree burns.

- DON'T ice a burn. Ice is too cold and might cause even more damage to the skin. Instead, soothe a burn by applying cool water.
- DON'T slather on butter. When the outer layers of your skin are gone, you're more vulnerable to infection, and butter can be loaded with bacteria.
- DON'T bandage the burn tightly. Instead, cover it with a loose, clean dressing so the burned area and any affected joints can move.
- DON'T mess with the blister. If a blister appears, your body has created its own bandage to protect itself.
- DO fill up on fluids to keep your skin hydrated and improve its ability to heal.

coffee grinder. Steep this mixture for 20 minutes. Strain. Pour it into your cool bath and soak.

Caffeine Addiction

Yes, coffee is an herb. But herbalists consider it the Jekyll and Hyde of the botanical world. Made from the roasted and ground seeds of the *Coffea arabica* plant, coffee—in moderation—perks you up, improves your reflexes, and helps you concentrate. It can also send your pulse and heartbeat racing, elevate blood pressure, trigger hot

- DO eat plenty of protein and vitamin C to help re-build collagen, a building block of skin tissue, and to speed healing.

- DO seek immediate medical care if the burn is ex-tremely tender, painful, swollen, and blistered; if it has pus, yellowish drainage, or a yellowish crust; if the area around the burn looks red or feels hot; or if you have signs of a fever.

- DO try this herbal remedy for minor burns from herbalist Rosemary Gladstar, director of the Sage Mountain Herbal Education Center in East Barre, Vermont. Blend one or two drops each of peppermint and lavender essential oils with 1 tablespoon of honey. Gently dab the mixture on the affected burn site. Loosely cover with a gauze wrap and leave on for a few hours or overnight. Reapply as needed until the skin heals. Peppermint and lavender first cool the burn and then take away the pain. Honey acts as a disinfectant, blocking germs from entering the wound.

flashes, and bring on jitters and headaches. And there is some controversial evidence indicating that consuming too much caffeine can aggravate the painful, but harmless, breast lumps sometimes referred to by doctors as fibro-cystic breast disease.

Although coffee is the first item to come to mind when we think of caffeine, its jolt is also found in some teas, colas, and chocolate. How much is safe? As a bench-mark, experts recommend no more than a 5-ounce cup or two of coffee a day, one 8-ounce cup of tea, or one 12-ounce can of soda.

Many of us consume much more than that. If you're ready to give up caffeine but you worry about losing that energizing zip—or if you're concerned about the headaches that can come with caffeine withdrawal—relax. Herbs can ease withdrawal symptoms. The real key to kicking the caffeine habit is to make a gradual shift by replacing caffeinated beverages with a drink that's flavorful and boosts your energy levels in a healthier way. Here's how.

Sip green tea. Start weaning yourself away from coffee by drinking green tea instead. This herbal tea contains 40 to 100 milligrams of caffeine per cup (the amount increases with steeping time)—about as much as coffee. But unlike coffee, green tea also contains polyphenols and catechins, compounds that protect your heart by lowering cholesterol. These substances also provide some protection against cancer and act as powerful antioxidants.

Brew a natural energy booster. Once you have successfully trimmed back your daily dose of caffeine, try this energizing tonic. Blend equal parts of chicory root, dandelion root, and milk thistle seed. Use 1 tablespoon of this mix per cup of boiling water. Steep for at least 5 minutes (10 to 15 is better). Chicory, dandelion, and milk thistle are thought by herbalists to stimulate your liver. They also assist your body in fighting stress.

Canker Sores

What is tiny, stays out of sight, and instantly ruins your enjoyment of even the finest meal? A canker sore.

Also called mouth ulcers, these recurrent, crater-shaped lesions can pop up almost anywhere on your tongue, inside your lips, or on the mucous membranes that line your cheeks.

What triggers a canker sore? Stress, nutritional deficiencies, tongue biting, bacteria, and highly acidic or salty foods are among the most common agents. Fortunately, most canker sores heal themselves within a week or so. You can shorten their natural course and keep yourself comfortable with these herbal healing strategies.

Rinse with echinacea. A little bit of echinacea goes a long way in healing canker sores, thanks to active constituents that boost the immune system. Try this mouth rinse: Add a dropperful or two of echinacea tincture to a glass of water. Two or three times a day, swish this rinse around in your mouth, then spit it out.

Try tea tree oil and water. Treat your canker sore naturally with a mouth rinse made from tea tree essential oil. This volatile oil from an Australian tree possesses antiseptic qualities. Simply add a few drops to a cup of water. Look for a tea tree oil product that contains 15 percent or less of cineole to avoid irritating your skin. Swish the rinse around in your mouth, then spit it out. Do not swallow the rinse.

Go for grapefruit power. Biting into a section of tart, acidic grapefruit would be torturous for anyone saddled with a canker sore. Yet, in the form of grapefruit seed extract, this fruit provides welcome relief. Grapefruit's sour powers outmuscle bacterial infections in your mouth.

Quell mouth pain by dabbing some grapefruit seed extract directly on the canker sore several times daily. As an added boost, add 5 drops to a glass of water and swish the solution around in your mouth three times a day.

Cervical Changes and Genital Warts

Name the most common sexually transmitted diseases these days, and you're sure to mention AIDS—and perhaps herpes, syphilis, or gonorrhea. But don't overlook the human papillomavirus (HPV), a virus that causes genital

> • *Herb at a Glance* •
> **Comfrey.** Good for reducing inflammation associated with bruises, sprains, and dislocations (topical application only)

warts, changes in cervical cells, and, if left untreated, even cervical cancer—often without detectable symptoms.

This highly contagious virus can infiltrate skin on the genitals or anus or invade the vaginal wall or the outer surface of the cervix. Transmitted through sexual contact with an infected partner, internal HPV infection offers no telltale signs; it can only be detected by a Pap test. There, the presence of HPV shows up as abnormal changes in cervical cells—changes that make these cells resemble cancer cells. Although cervical changes (also called cervical dysplasia) are not cancerous, this condition must be taken very seriously because it can develop into cancer if not treated in time.

By contrast, you may see or feel external genital warts, also caused by HPV. If these swollen bumps appear on your genitals or anus, they may itch. But if they appear inside your cervix, genital warts are flat and symptom-free—even though they can be caused by the most virulent strains of HPV.

You can reduce your risk of contracting HPV by using condoms during sexual intercourse. It's also important to have an annual gynecological exam, including a Pap test, to detect the presence of warts or cervical changes. If HPV is discovered, get prompt treatment; never try to treat genital warts or cervical changes on your own.

If you would like to go the natural route, work with an experienced physician who is well-versed in herbal medicine. Herbal therapy, managed by a good doctor, can help prevent the progression of the disease, reverse cervical changes, and prevent recurrence. A doctor will also know when you should have a biopsy or even have precancerous cells removed. Along with doctor-supervised natural therapies, you can take steps at home to soothe discomfort and boost your immune system during treatment. Here are a few herbal strategies to consider.

Bolster immunity with garlic and a saintly herb. Garlic and St. John's wort are among the leading immune-enhancing herbs that can tackle an invading virus. Experts recommend taking two to four capsules of garlic daily and 4 dropperfuls of St. John's wort tincture in the morning and evening every other day.

Bathe in oatmeal. Soothe wart-related genital itching with Aveeno bath treatment. You can purchase it in any drugstore. This product contains a finely powdered oatmeal called colloidal oatmeal, known to ease itching. It also won't clog your bathtub drain.

Smooth on an herbal soother. Apply a cream or salve containing calendula, plantain leaf, aloe, or chamomile to your vulva in the morning and evening as needed. These herbal creams stop the irritation, redness, and itching of genital warts. Select creams that do not contain perfumes or essential oils that might irritate tender mucous membranes. These creams can be purchased in health food stores or through mail order.

Chapped Lips

Every day, indoors and out, the climate attacks our lips. Your lips are fragile: While a pigment called melanin protects the rest of the skin on your body from the elements, your lips lack this weather guard. So it's up to you to provide some dependable protection against assault. Try these herbal helpers for moist, pain-free lips.

Moisturize with castor oil. Purchase a small bottle of castor oil at the drugstore. Dab a few drops on your lips to soothe the sting caused by cracking. This inexpensive oil coats your lips and offers a thick lacquer of shine.

Stir in skin-friendly eucalyptus. For really chapped and sore lips, add 10 drops of eucalyptus essential oil to a 2-ounce bottle of castor oil. Dab on lips as needed. Eucalyptus gives the castor oil a skin-healing boost.

Look for a healing balm. Herbalists recommend the herbs lavender, calendula, plantain, nettle, chamomile, and comfrey to soothe chapped lips and promote healing. Check out health food stores to find a ready-made, all-natural lip balm that contains one or more of these healing herbs. The best balms are made with olive oil and beeswax, which herbalists recommend to moisturize and protect lips.

Colds and Flu

Herbal therapies have unique powers to boost your immune system so that it can better fight off the hundreds of different cold and flu viruses just waiting to invade your body and reproduce by the billions in your nose, throat, and lungs.

These invaders strike most often in winter. During this peak season, we're more likely to come in contact with nasty viruses because we spend more time indoors with other folks who may already be nursing a respiratory or digestive ailment. Then simply touching something—a doorknob, telephone, or anything that has been handled, sneezed at, or coughed on by a sick person within the previous 24 hours—heightens your own risk.

Beyond boosting immunity, botanical strategies can also help knock out a cold or flu in its early stages, and they can minimize symptoms at any point, bringing you relief. Here's how to take advantage of their powers.

Stockpile echinacea. At the first sign of illness, take a dose of echinacea, long hailed among Native Americans as the classic cold-and-flu warrior. Scientists say echinacea activates the production of two proteins in your body—interferon and properdin—that battle viruses.

Follow the package dosage directions for echinacea tinctures, capsules, or tea. But be sure to take it often: every hour or two for the first day, then three times a day until your symptoms have subsided. Continue taking echinacea

---

THE HERBAL KITCHEN

Stinging Nettle Tea for Colds and Coughs

Nettle leaves make a delicious tea and contain a variety of nutrients, says herbalist Rosemary Gladstar, director of the Sage Mountain Herbal Education Center in East Barre, Vermont. So the next time you have a sore throat, upset stomach, cold, cough, or congestion, try Gladstar's spinachy-tasting stinging nettle tea recipe as a nice complement to other decongesting remedies.

1 cup water
1 teaspoon dried stinging nettle leaves (see note)
1 teaspoon honey (optional)

Bring the water to a boil in a saucepan. Add the nettle, cover, and boil for 20 minutes. Strain out the nettle. Sweeten the tea with the honey, if desired.

Note: If fresh nettle is available, use 2 teaspoons of the leaves. Wear gloves to pick young, tender, light green leaves from their stems, and avoid the plant's stinging hairs. Discard the stems and thoroughly wash the leaves.

for about 3 more days once you're feeling well. One note: If you use echinacea tincture "straight" (without water), you may notice a slight numbness in your mouth immediately after taking a dose. This sensation is harmless and short-lived, and it's a sign that you have genuine echinacea.

Heap on the garlic. Crushed or mashed, garlic is an antiviral herb that helps take the punch out of a cold. If you're worried about bad breath, take enteric-coated garlic capsules in 300-milligram dosages three times a day for as long as your cold symptoms last. Then breathe a sweet-smelling sigh of relief. If you don't mind garlic breath, eat several raw cloves a day—chopped and added to salads, soups, or entrées—until your symptoms subside.

Try a berry good virus fighter. Elderberry contains two compounds that prevent flu viruses from invading respiratory tract cells. Studies have shown that flu sufferers who used an elderberry product showed significant relief of fever, muscle aches, and other symptoms within 24 hours. Read the label for proper dosage amounts.

Soothe aches and nausea with ginger tea. Ginger is well-regarded by herbalists for its stomach-soothing and ache-relieving abilities. For nausea and muscle aches, drink a cup of ginger tea up to four times a day. Simmer 1 teaspoon of grated fresh ginger and 1 cup of water in a covered pot for 10 minutes. Then strain and sip.

Congestion

You draw air in and out of your lungs automatically 23,000 times a day. Each inhalation brings in the fresh oxygen that every cell in your body needs. But it's also an open invitation to airborne dust, pollen, and tobacco smoke as well as cold and flu viruses, all of which can leave you feeling stuffed up.

Dust and smoke act like sandpaper, scraping and irritating the delicate membranes in your nose and sinuses. Cold and flu viruses can also irritate these membranes, causing them to swell. This blocks sinus passages so that they can't drain. The result? Congestion—that all-stopped-up, can't-breathe feeling.

The next time you are saddled with a stuffy nose and want relief, turn to these safe herbal remedies, which offer comfort without side effects.

Reduce stuffiness with herbal steam. The moist steam rising from hot herbal tea can help break up nasal and chest congestion caused by colds, flu, smoke, or allergies. Select pungent herbs like peppermint, ginger, yarrow, thyme, or lemon verbena. Add a handful to a pot of boiling water. Then turn off the heat and place the pot on a trivet on the kitchen counter. Cover your head with a large towel and lean over the pan. Keep your head about 12 inches above the pot. Slowly breathe in the vapors alternately through your nose and mouth for about 10 minutes. You can bring your face closer as the steam cools.

The hot vapors from these herbs help liquefy mucus, fight germs, and open passageways in the nose, sinuses, and chest.

Unclog gingerly. To reduce inflammation and open clogged nasal passages, natural healers rely on ginger tea—in part because of its rich zinc content. Finely chop a thin slice of fresh ginger and add it to 1 cup of water. Boil gently in a covered pan for 10 to 15 minutes. Strain and add a squeeze of lemon or a spoonful of honey, if desired.

> • *Herb at a Glance* •
> **Dandelion.** Good for stimulating the production of bile, which aids in the digestion of fat

Lay on the onion. To help break up chest congestion, dice two onions and place the pieces in a pan. Cook gently with a little oil until the onion bits are transparent. Cool, then lay the pieces across your chest. Place plastic wrap over the onions (use a piece that fully covers the onions). Put a warm towel or warm water bottle wrapped in a cloth on top of the plastic wrap. Leave the onions on your chest for about 30 minutes.

The secret behind this old-fashioned remedy is the essential oils in the onions. They're believed to help fight any infection related to the congestion. Herbalists say onion also stimulates bloodflow, which they believe helps your body break up congestion and move waste material away.

Constipation

Constipation is simply any deviation from normal that makes your bowels more sluggish. The best strategy for getting your bowels back on track is to adjust your eating plan. Consume at least five servings of fruits and vegetables and two servings of whole grains a day. And drink at least eight 8-ounce glasses of water. Of course, to be on the safe side, you should see your doctor if you notice any sudden change in your bowel movements, including the size, color, or consistency or the presence of blood.

In addition to improving your diet, try the following herbs to gently coax your bowels back into action.

First, try flaxseed. Grind a teaspoon of whole flaxseed in a coffee grinder and stir it into an 8-ounce glass of water or juice. Sip one of these flax cocktails with each meal until your constipation subsides. Flaxseed is rich in fiber.

Prompt faster action with dandelion. This common "weed" contains bitter compounds that can help stimulate contractions of the colon and move stools along. It is also thought to stimulate bile flow. Herbalists recommend using 1 to 3 dropperfuls of dandelion root tincture in ¼ cup of water. (A dropperful is about 15 drops.) Drink slowly, savoring each mouthful for about a minute.

Soften stubborn stools with licorice and prunes. When all else fails, call on the bowel-loosening team of licorice root and prunes. Make a licorice-prune tea by simmering ½ teaspoon of licorice root in ½ cup of water for 2 minutes. Remove from the heat and steep for 15 minutes. Strain out the root and soak three stewed prunes in the tea for a few hours. Eat the prunes and drink the tea (have them cold or slightly warm) before going to bed, to give stools a needed nudge. You should experience relief by morning.

Coughs

It's very hard to stop a cough. And for good reason, you shouldn't even try. Coughing is a natural reflex designed to expel excess mucus from your lungs.

Still, a cough may erupt at the most inopportune times, and a persistent cough can inflame your throat and even make your chest hurt. For stubborn coughs that don't disappear after 2 weeks—or that bring up discolored phlegm (not clear or whitish)—see your doctor. Otherwise, try these natural ways to silence that hacking.

Summon horehound to the rescue. For aggravating coughs, suck on cough drops containing horehound, natural healers suggest. This herb acts as an antispasmodic, soothing muscle spasms that produce coughs, as well as a decongestant.

Give a cough the slip with slippery elm. To calm a persistent cough and soothe your irritated throat, herbalists recommend slippery elm throat lozenges. Native Americans relied on this herb for cough relief because it contains large amounts of mucilage, which acts as a mild cough suppressant. Herbalists recommend taking slippery elm in throat lozenges instead of tea because the lozenges provide a steady stream of mucilage to coat your throat.

Call for tea thyme. Relax airway muscles and clear up congestion by drinking thyme tea three times a day for up to 3 days. Thyme acts as an expectorant and relieves bronchial spasms triggered by excessive coughing. To make the tea, pour ¾ cup of freshly boiled water over 2 teaspoons of fresh thyme leaves (or 1 teaspoon dried thyme). Cover and steep for 10 minutes, then strain. Let the tea cool before drinking it. After 3 days, stop this remedy and see your doctor if your coughing and irritated throat do not improve.

Clear up congestion with elecampane. For coughing accompanied by thick congestion, herbalists suggest elecampane root tea. Pour 1 cup of cold water over 1 teaspoon of chopped elecampane root in a saucepan. Simmer for about 20 minutes, strain, then drink the warm tea. Have up to three cups of this tea a day while you have a cough. Elecampane root expels mucus and dries out mucous membranes. Plus, it contains mucilage, so it soothes your irritated throat. This herb is bitter tasting, so you may need to add some honey to sweeten it a bit.

Cuts and Scrapes

Your skin is prepared for everyday cuts and scrapes. After an injury, your body's natural repair team quickly arrives at the scene to protect against infection and rebuild damaged cell layers. You can boost your body's innate healing powers by following some commonsense rules about caring for injured skin and by choosing skin-friendly botanicals to help protect and mend minor wounds.

How do you tell if your cut is more than a minor mishap? If the cut is large (more than ½ inch long) or deep into the yellow, fatty layer of your skin, you need to see a doctor for stitches. Stitches help the cut heal faster and reduce your chance of scarring. You may need an antibiotic if the cut area is red, tender, or oozing pus or if you have a fever.

For a minor cut or scrape, begin by cleaning out any dirt to reduce the risk of infection. Doctors suggest cleaning cuts and scrapes three times a day. Plain old soap and water works well, or you can try one of the following herbal washes to fight bacteria and swelling, protect sensitive, unhealed skin, and promote the birth of healthy new skin cells.

Prepare antiseptic herbs in advance. Get ready for the next cut or scrape by making this easy herbal antiseptic formula ahead of time. Mix ½ ounce each of the following tinctures (sometimes labeled as extracts): calendula, echinacea, Oregon grape root, and St. John's wort.

Store this mixture in a 2-ounce dark glass bottle with a dropper in the lid. Mark the date on the bottle. This homemade first-aid tincture has a shelf life of about a year. When the need arises to clean a cut or scrape, combine equal parts of the antiseptic mixture and sterile water (available in most drugstores).

Cleanse with myrrh. You can ease the pain of cuts and scrapes and fight infection with myrrh, an astringent that prompts healing. Myrrh is a reddish brown resin that flows from the bark of a species of shrubs and small trees in Africa and south-western Asia. Herbalists recommend dissolving 1 teaspoon of myrrh powder in 1 cup of warm water. Then use that liquid mix to wash out a cut right away.

> • *Herb at a Glance* •
>
> **Echinacea.** Good for combating colds, flu, infections, slow-healing wounds, and inflamed skin conditions

Double up on the calendula. To promote healing and help clean up any residual debris caught beneath the skin, herbalists suggest calendula, used two ways. First, mix 25 drops of calendula tincture in 4 ounces of sterile water and apply directly to the wound as needed. Then apply calendula ointment directly to the wound or dab some on a bandage and cover.

In the late 1800s, American cowboys used calendula to stop bleeding and to heal bullet wounds. Researchers have found that this herb can also decrease swelling and spur growth of new skin cells.

Quell pain with St. John's wort. When scrapes cause pain, an infused oil of St. John's wort works better than aspirin, say some alternative medicine experts. Dip a cotton swab in the oil and apply directly to the cut.

Dandruff

Those annoying white flakes that shower down from your scalp onto your shoulders are more than an inconvenience. They're skin cells on the move.

In dandruff-free hair, new skin cells migrate to the surface of the scalp and shed without notice every 21 days. Dandruff results when these cells reach the surface in half the time. As a result, cells build up on your scalp in clumps before they're shed. When they do shed, they look like a snow flurry in your hair and on your clothing.

Oily hair and yeast infections of the scalp also prompt your head to shed dead skin cells in large clumps. Seasonal changes that dry out your scalp only make matters worse.

If dandruff makes your scalp red and very itchy and persists despite at-home treatment, see your doctor. You may need treatment for a fungal infection or for seborrheic dermatitis, an inflammation of the oil glands. For mild dandruff, natural healers suggest botanical remedies that work on the scalp itself as well as remedies that are taken internally. Combined, they help control itching and flaking.

Cleanse from the inside with burdock. Some herbalists believe that dandruff is a sign of an unhealthy liver, a signal that this vital organ isn't processing waste material from the blood effectively. They say you can attack dandruff from the inside out by improving your liver and cleansing your blood with burdock tea.

Prepare burdock tea with 1 to 2 teaspoons of root per cup of boiling water. Fresh grated root is best, but it is available for harvesting only from late spring through early fall. Dried, organic burdock roots are more readily available year-round from health food stores. Boil these roots for 15 to 20 minutes, then strain the tea and drink up to three cups a day. You should see fewer flakes within a month.

Vanquish flakes with an herbal rinse. Stop itching and slow the buildup of white scalp flakes by rinsing your hair with this anti-dandruff formula. Take a handful each of dried nettle tops, dried calendula flowers, and dried rosemary and place these herbs in a 2-quart glass jar. Cover the herbs with a quart of organic apple-cider vinegar. Close the jar and let it stand at least 2 weeks (ideally, 1 month) before straining.

Use 1 cup to rinse your hair after every shampoo and leave it in. If you find that it's too strong, you can use 1 to 2 tablespoons in 1 cup of water.

Boost scalp health with a witch hazel splash. Apple-cider vinegar mixed with skin-friendly herbs and witch hazel helps maintain the natural acid balance of your scalp, which will improve general scalp health. Create an herbal splash by infusing any combination of calendula, plantain, and comfrey in apple-cider vinegar.

Use a quart jar half-packed with dried herbs or fully packed with fresh herbs. Cover with the vinegar. Steep it for 3 to 6 weeks, then strain. For every 3 cups of vinegar, add 1 cup of distilled water and 2 tablespoons of witch hazel. When you're ready to use it, mix about 2 tablespoons into a pint of water for an after-shampoo rinse.

Dental Health

How can you maintain a healthy, attractive smile? No news here. Brush and floss daily and report faithfully for dental checkups twice a year.

You can further guard your smile by watching what you eat. Food and drinks loaded with sugar or acid (such as lemon juice) can cause plaque buildup, tooth enamel erosion, cavities, and tooth decay. Beyond these basic strategies, however, herbalists offer botanical remedies for a host of common dental concerns.

Prevent plaque with bloodroot. To keep sticky dental plaque from adhering to your teeth, select toothpastes and mouthwashes that contain bloodroot. Studies have shown that dental-care products containing this herb can reduce plaque buildup on teeth within as little as 8 days. Bloodroot contains sanguinarine, an alkaloid that chemically binds to dental plaque and keeps it from sticking to your teeth. Viadent, a popular mouthwash and toothpaste brand, contains bloodroot.

Trade diet soda for tea. To prevent cavities, switch your drink of choice from diet soda to herbal tea. A diet soda with a lemon twist may save you some calories, but it eats away at your tooth enamel. Green and black teas, by contrast, contain a generous amount of tooth-preserving fluoride. Four cups of tea per day—hot or cold—give you all the fluoride you need.

Sweeten with sugar-free licorice. Need a bit of sweetness for your herbal tea? Licorice is a natural sugar-free sweetener that contains two tooth-protecting ingredients: glycyrrhizin, which kills bacteria, and indole, which prevents tooth decay. For a sweet taste, skip the table sugar and brew your green or black tea with a pinch of dried licorice root.

Depression

Everyone sings the blues from time to time. A relationship ends. A job promotion falls through. That down-in-the-dumps feeling usually fades within a few days. But if it lingers for 2 weeks or more, it may be depression.

Research suggests that genes and biochemistry as well as personal history and recent life circumstances contribute to depression. It's an illness—not a character flaw—that can run in families. Hormonal changes just before menstruation and after pregnancy also appear to make some women more prone to feeling depressed. Certain prescription drugs and chronic illnesses trigger bouts of depression, too. Whatever the cause, the signs of depression can appear in every aspect of your life. You may feel guilty, angry, or powerless. You may withdraw from others, overeat, lose your appetite, or find it difficult to sleep at night.

Once you recognize that you're depressed, you can begin seeking relief. For severe depression (if, for example, you're having trouble functioning in your daily life or you have thoughts of suicide), see a doctor immediately.

Mild depression, on the other hand, may respond well to self-care with herbal remedies. Next time you get a case of the blues, give these botanical mood lifters a try.

Depend on nature's Prozac. Nature's top healer in the battle against depression is St. John's wort. Although this common, yellow-flowered plant has gained lots of attention in recent years, natural healers have actually relied upon it for thousands of years. And European researchers have concluded that St. John's wort works as

> • *Herb at a Glance* •
> **Eucalyptus.** Good for
> bronchitis and throat
> inflammations

well as standard antide-
pressants such as Prozac
for treating mild to mod-
erate levels of depres-
sion—without the side
effects of drugs.

This herb appears to work in several ways at once: by
normalizing levels of cortisol, a substance that helps your
body deal with stress, and by activating the secretion of
dopamine, a pleasure hormone.

St. John's wort comes in capsules, tinctures, and teas.
Check with your doctor or a qualified herbalist to select
the best form for you.

If you choose capsules, slowly build the dosage to one
300-milligram capsule three times a day. For tinctures,
take 4 dropperfuls in a little water in the morning and
3 in the evening. Some experts suggest looking for standardized St. John's wort products that contain 0.3 percent
hypericin, one of the herb's active ingredients. Give this
herb at least 4 to 6 weeks to take effect.

Soak in mood-lifting scents. For hundreds of years,
healers have noted that the fragrance of certain herbs has
the power to dispel a blue mood. Today, some herbalists and
researchers believe that essential-oil fragrances may have an
effect on the brain that is similar to that of antidepressants.
Try it for yourself by adding this uplifting fragrance blend to
your next bath. Combine 2 ounces of almond oil, 10 drops
each of bergamot and petitgrain essential oils, 3 drops of
rose geranium essential oil, and 1 drop of neroli essential oil
(it's expensive, so you can leave it out if you'd like). Pour
the mixture into a tubful of warm water and soak.

By adding an additional 2 ounces of almond oil, you can
turn this recipe into a fragrance to dab onto your wrists.

Sip the "happy herbs." Try a three-herb tea that can lift
your spirits in three ways. It contains calcium-rich oat-

straw, which strengthens the nervous system; lemon balm, which has a traditional reputation as the "gladdening herb"; and damiana, which is known in the Southwest as the happy herb. Damiana also is thought to balance hormone levels. Combine equal parts of all three, then use 1 teaspoon to 1 tablespoon per cup of boiling water. Steep for 5 minutes, strain, and sip one to three cups a day.

Root out anger with dandelion. For depression that's more a case of unexpressed anger, down some dandelion root tea. It seems to help some people recognize and express withheld anger that can lead to feelings of numbness and depression, say some herbalists.

Use 1 tablespoon of dandelion root per cup of boiling water, steep or simmer for 10 to 20 minutes, then strain and sip. Have 2 to 3 cups a day for best results.

Diabetes

When your body's fuel-delivery system is working right, carbohydrates smoothly convert into glucose, the body's chief source of energy. This simple sugar is then channeled through your bloodstream. It prompts your pancreas to secrete insulin, the hormone that ushers sugar into every cell in your body.

For people with diabetes, glucose can't enter cells efficiently. Either the pancreas doesn't produce enough insulin or cells resist the insulin's attempts to deliver sugar—or both happen at once. Uncontrolled, diabetes can cause serious, sometimes fatal, complications. Sugar can build up in your bloodstream, damaging your blood vessels, nerves, eyes, and kidneys. Wounds take longer to heal and circulation slows.

Doctors often prescribe insulin, to be taken either orally or by injection, depending on the type of diabetes you have. Type 1 diabetes requires daily insulin injections to maintain safe blood sugar levels. Non-insulin-dependent diabetes—type 2—can be controlled through a combination of diet, exercise, and oral medications that boost the effect of your body's insulin. Maintaining a healthy weight is also important.

While you should never stop taking insulin as prescribed by your physician, you can incorporate the following herbs into your daily routine to help regulate your blood sugar levels and possibly lessen the impact of diabetes. Be sure to talk with your doctor before adding these herbs to your treatment plan, and continue monitoring your blood sugar levels carefully. Report any change to your doctor promptly.

Spice up your tea. Add a pinch or two each of bay leaf, cinnamon, cloves, and turmeric to a pot of black tea. Steep for 10 minutes. Pour over some ice in a glass and drink. Research shows that these spices help the body use insulin more efficiently.

Improve sugar stability with ginseng. People with type 2 diabetes may gain greater control of their blood sugar levels by taking ginseng. A Finnish study found that people with diabetes who took 200 milligrams of ginseng every day had more stable blood sugar levels.

Spoon up a special bean soup. To help maintain blood sugar at desired levels, try this fiber-fortified bean soup. In a large pan, bring 2 cups of water and one unpeeled onion (quartered) to a boil over medium heat. Add one 16-ounce can of kidney beans (rinsed and drained), one small diced carrot, ½ cup peanuts, ½ teaspoon fenugreek seeds, two bay leaves, four chopped garlic cloves, and a dash each of ground cinnamon, ground cloves, and turmeric.

Bring to a simmer, then cover and cook for 30 minutes. Remove the onion pieces with a slotted spoon, and peel off and discard the skins. Lightly mash the onions with a fork and return to the saucepan. Discard the bay leaves. This recipe makes four servings.

Research has shown that beans, which are high in soluble fiber, help balance sugar levels. Onions, especially the skins, are rich in quercetin, which has been found to help with eye problems associated with diabetes. Fenugreek contains six blood sugar–regulating compounds. Bay leaves may help your body use insulin more efficiently. And garlic may lower insulin resistance.

Diarrhea

Diarrhea keeps you on the run—right to the bathroom. Those loose, watery stools are your body's way of saying "out with the bad."

Diagnosing diarrhea is easy. There's nothing subtle about the symptoms. Determining what triggers a sudden attack of the runs can be trickier. It could be a bacterial or viral infection, sudden stress, too much caffeine, or eating foods to which you're sensitive. All of these can irritate your intestines to the point of diarrhea.

Most diarrhea lasts no more than a few days, but during that time you could become dehydrated and lose valuable nutrients your body needs. And, of course, it's hard to maintain your day-to-day life when you're always dashing to the bathroom.

Before turning to any remedy—herbal or over-the-counter—scrutinize your eating habits and stress levels. People who consume high-fiber diets (lots of fruits, vegetables, and whole grains) and keep stress under control rarely have diarrhea. But if you need immediate relief or if you still have minor diarrhea after altering your diet, try these herbal diarrhea stoppers. Of course, contact your doctor if diarrhea persists for more than 2 days or if you see blood in your stool.

Call on cinnamon for emergency relief. Frequent bouts of diarrhea can lead to dehydration because your body is losing valuable fluids. To "dry up" bowels quickly, make some cinnamon tea. Cinnamon is a natural astringent that will curb the loss of fluids. To make the tea, mix 1 tablespoon of dried powdered cinnamon bark into 1 cup of hot water. Steep 10 to 15 minutes.

Curb the runs with blueberries. If you're on the road and unable to make a pot of healing herbal tea to stop diarrhea, natural healers suggest this take-anywhere remedy. Keep a bag of dried blueberries within easy reach. Chew and swallow 3 tablespoons for relief. Don't substitute fresh blueberries; they may actually cause diarrhea. Dried blueberries contain astringent tannins that reduce intestinal inflammation and help shield the stomach wall from toxins. The dried berries also contain absorbent pectins, which can reduce fluid loss.

Soothe with slippery elm. Slippery elm bark is a popular diarrhea fighter among herbalists because it contains slippery mucilage, which soothes irritated intestines. Take a few spoonfuls of slippery elm powder and blend in enough honey to create a thick dough. Roll the mixture into small balls. Finish by dusting the balls with a little more slippery elm powder. At the first sign of diarrhea, let a ball dissolve slowly in your mouth, and repeat as necessary. Store the rest of the balls in a closed container in the refrigerator and use as needed. (To keep the balls indefinitely, dry them in a very low oven—just the pilot light will work—for a few hours or in the sun for a few days.)

Replenish lost nutrients with a multi-herb tea. Important minerals, including potassium, chloride, and sodium, are washed from your body during bouts of diarrhea. These nutrients help your body regulate the flow of water across mucous membranes. You can restore them, herbalists say, by drinking a tea made with one or all of the following herbs: alfalfa, nettle, red raspberry leaves, and red clover. Use up to 1 tablespoon of dried herbs per cup of hot water. Steep about 15 minutes and strain the herbs. Then drink up to 5 cups a day until your symptoms retreat.

Dry and Sun-Damaged Hair

Dry hair looks dull and lifeless. It may stick straight out like the bristles on a broom, lie limply, or frizz up. Desert-dry tresses simply won't do your bidding.

What steals the shine and body? Blame the weather, which robs hair of moisture. But don't stop there. Our own primping also takes its toll, thanks to bleaching, coloring, straightening, perming, and using blow-dryers and curling irons.

Any of these can fry your crowning glory by damaging the outer layer of each hair shaft, called the cuticle. The cuticle consists of cells that overlap, sort of like shingles on a roof. Healthy cuticle cells lie flat, holding in moisture and reflecting light. This kind of hair feels healthy and looks shiny. But when cuticle cells get roughed up by intense heat or harsh chemicals, the hair shaft loses moisture and dulls.

These natural remedies should work beautifully to restore your hair's natural luster.

Make hair shimmer with essential oils. Add body and shine to dry and sun-damaged hair with this easy deep-conditioning treatment using essential oils. Take ¼ cup of olive, jojoba, or sweet almond oil and add 10 drops of lavender or rosemary essential oil. For

• *Herb at a Glance* •

Fennel. Good for easing painful gas and stimulating the appetite and digestion thick, heavy hair, coconut oil works best. Wet your hair and rub in the oil mix until your hair is thoroughly coated. Cover with a shower cap and a warm towel for 30 minutes. Then shampoo twice.

Concoct an herbal conditioner. Moisturize dry hair with an easy-to-make botanical conditioner. Combine 1 teaspoon of each of the following dried herbs: burdock root, calendula flowers, chamomile flowers, lavender flowers, and rosemary leaves. Pour 1 pint of freshly boiled water over the herbs. Allow them to steep for 30 minutes. Strain the mixture and add 1 tablespoon of vinegar. Wash your hair with a moisturizing shampoo (one that contains natural oils, glycerin, honey, or amino acids) and rinse. Then pour this herbal conditioner over your hair. Don't rinse.

Lubricate the ends, fragrantly. For dry, wispy hair, a few drops of sandalwood or rosemary essential oil works wonders on flyaway ends without leaving a greasy residue— and it smells great! Put two drops of either oil on your fingertips and massage it into the ends of your hair.

Moisturize from the inside out with evening primrose oil. Evening primrose oil is rich in essential fatty acids, which are vital to healthy hair and skin. Herbalists suggest taking one to three 250-milligram capsules of this herb one to three times a day. You can substitute flaxseed oil capsules, which also contain essential fatty acids.

Dry Skin

Your skin is vulnerable to all sorts of moisture-robbing conditions, including sun, wind, and winter cold, as well as the dry air in heated and air-conditioned rooms. These forces suppress oil production, leading to itchy, flaky skin.

You can fight dry-skin foes naturally. Start by drinking at least eight 8-ounce glasses of water daily to moisturize from the inside out. Also make sure your diet includes oils high in monounsaturated fats, such as olive and canola oil. In addition, wash with a water-soluble cleansing cream instead of soap. Most soaps dry out skin. And avoid facial toners that contain alcohol, another moisture stealer.

THE HERBAL KITCHEN

Bath Salts

Tap water often contains calcium and magnesium, making it "hard." Hard water can leave your skin dull and rough. Bath salts counteract these minerals to silken and soften the water. They also help to remove body oils and perspiration.

To make your own bath salts, follow this simple recipe created by Mindy Green, a founding and professional member of the American Herbalists Guild and director of educational services for the Herb Research Foundation in Boulder, Colorado. It takes only easy-to-find ingredients, including borax, a natural mineral salt that is used as a laundry detergent.

  2 cups borax
  ½ cup sea salt
  ½ cup baking soda
  ½ teaspoon essential oil (see note)

In a bowl, mix the borax, sea salt, and baking soda. Stir in the essential oil. Use ¼ to ½ cup of the bath salts per bath. For muscular aches and pains, add ½ cup of Epsom salts to the recipe. Store the mixture in a wide-mouth, dark-colored glass jar.

Note: Suggested essential oils are neroli, marjoram, or lavender for relaxation; rosemary, juniper, or eucalyptus for stimulation and muscle relaxation; and geranium or orange for stress relief.

If your skin is still dry and flaky, try these gentle botanical remedies to restore a healthy, moist glow.

Sink into a tub of oats. If your entire body feels dry and irritated, an oatmeal bath can ditch the itch. The gentle cleansing power of oats seems tailor-made for dry skin. Their slippery quality soothes, moisturizes, and heals. To prepare an oatmeal bath, place ½ to 1 cup of old-fashioned rolled oats in a muslin bag or a handkerchief closed securely with a rubber band. Place the bag in the tub and run warm water. Don't pour oats out of the box into the tub or they'll clog the drain.

Alternately, you can soothe dry skin with Aveeno bath treatment, which is available in any drugstore. This product contains a finely powdered oatmeal called colloidal oatmeal, known to ease itching. It also won't clog your bathtub drain.

Switch to an herbal cleanser. If you have a dry complexion and need a soap substitute that won't rob moisture from your skin, natural healers recommend this easy-to-make botanical cleanser. In a bottle with a lid, blend 2 ounces of aloe vera gel, 1 teaspoon of grapeseed oil, 1 teaspoon of glycerin, ½ teaspoon of grapefruit seed extract, 8 drops of sandalwood essential oil, and 4 drops of rosemary essential oil. Shake well before each use. Apply this herbal cleanser with cotton balls, then rinse.

Blend a moisturizing mask. Soothe dry skin and protect against infection by applying this calendula-and-cream facial mask. Combine ¼ cup of whipping cream, ½ teaspoon of olive oil, 2 tablespoons of mashed ripe avocado, and 1 teaspoon each of calendula petals and lavender flowers. Let this mixture stand for 5 minutes to allow the liquid to soak up the herbs. Then whip by hand or in a food processor. Slather the mask on clean skin and leave it in place for at least 5 minutes. The cream, oil, and avocado in this mask provide much-needed moisture, while the herbs add skin-healing properties. (If a ripe avocado is hard to find, skip it.)

Earaches

It aches, it throbs, it stabs you from the inside out, and you can't even rub it to make it feel better.

When you experience intense, lasting pain in your ear, something has usually gone awry deep in the Eustachian tube—the pencil-thin canal that runs from the back of your nasal passage to your ear.

Sometimes an invading bacterium or virus causes inflammation and fluid buildup in this narrow passageway. Colds, allergies, and sore throats can also bring on the kind of ear congestion that causes discomfort and muffled hearing.

Treating an earache is not always a do-it-yourself proposition. If it's sudden and intense or accompanied by dizziness, a fever above 101°F, or discharge from your ear, see your doctor at once. Severe ear infections can cause your eardrum to burst.

For less severe earaches, however, herbalists choose botanical remedies that can numb the pain as well as help your body knock out the infection-causing virus or bacterium. These herbs also strengthen your immune system to keep ear infections from making unwelcome comebacks.

Calm aches with St. John's wort oil. For extremely achy ears, St. John's wort helps stop pain by acting as an anti-inflammatory that soothes irritated nerves in the ear canal. This herb also helps fight viruses. Mix a solution of one part St. John's wort infused oil and one part mullein flower infused

> • *Herb at a Glance* •
> **Garlic.** Good for bacterial and fungal infections, digestive ailments, and high blood pressure

oil. (Mullein oil has antimicrobial properties.) You can purchase or order infused oils from health food stores. Don't confuse them with essential oils; they're not the same. Put about 3 drops of this mix into the affected ear and cover with a cotton ball. Reapply the drops every 6 to 8 hours, using a fresh cotton ball.

Gain relief with garlic. According to some herbalists, ear infections are no match for the antibiotic properties of garlic oil. For more ache-easing power, combine equal parts garlic and mullein flower infused oils. Put 4 drops of this mix into the achy ear and cover with a cotton ball. Reapply the drops every 4 to 6 hours as needed, using a fresh cotton ball each time.

Fight back with echinacea. Echinacea, also known as coneflower, may give your immune system a boost and battle infection. Steep 1 teaspoon of dried echinacea in a cup of boiling water for about 10 minutes. Strain and sip. Or add a dropperful of echinacea tincture to juice or tea. Drink either beverage three times a day until your earache goes away.

Eczema

Just what is that scaly rash that has been driving you crazy lately? Is it serious? Will it ever go away? If it began as a reaction to stress, temperature extremes, or even scratchy clothing, then you may have eczema.

This skin condition often runs in families. Everything from emotional turmoil to extreme air temperatures to allergies can trigger an outbreak. So can extreme sensitivity to common foods like dairy products. In severe cases, eczema makes the skin thicken, blister, and crack, especially around the folds at your neck, elbows, and knees. Anyone with a case this bad should see a doctor.

Eczema can be soothed by keeping your skin constantly moist. Have a moisturizer handy at work and at home. It's also smart to rule out possible foods that might be making matters worse. A simple diet change could bring relief. Then rely on these herbal remedies to feel even better.

Pamper with slippery elm. Soothe itchy, inflamed skin rashes with an herbal paste. Mix slippery elm powder with enough water to form a thin paste. Apply the paste to the affected skin and leave it in place until it's dry—usually an hour or less. Rinse gently with water and pat your skin dry with a clean towel. Do this three times a day.

Slippery elm contains mucilage, which is known to moisturize, heal, and soothe skin.

Ditch the itch with evening primrose. You can soothe an eczema rash with evening primrose oil, an herb containing essential fatty acids that reduce inflammation. Take two to four 500-milligram capsules three times a day for best results.

Battle bacteria with goldenseal. For eczema that becomes infected, herbalists recommend goldenseal. Combine one part goldenseal tincture with three parts warm water. Soak a clean cloth in the mixture and apply it to the rash for 15 to 20 minutes. Reapply this antimicrobial wash four or five times a day. Goldenseal contains berberine, a substance that fights bacterial infections, redness, and inflammation.

Endometriosis

It's menstruation gone crazy. When you have endometriosis, heavy bleeding, sharp pain, and nausea can complicate your monthly periods. It can also inflict you with interrupted sleep, fatigue, depression, and infertility.

Endometriosis occurs when tissue from the lining of the uterus—the endometrium—migrates and grows on the

---
• *Herb at a Glance* •

Ginger. Good for motion
sickness, nausea,
and menstrual cramps

---

ovaries, bowel, bladder, or
other internal organs. This
tissue expands, then sheds
just as the normal uterine
lining does during the
course of the menstrual
cycle. But since it's not in the right place, it causes pain
and other problems instead of simply leaving the body as
menstrual blood.

Medical experts don't know exactly why about 1 in
every 10 American women develops endometriosis, but
they theorize that an abundance of the hormone estrogen
can heighten the risk. Heredity and stress as well as environmental pollutants are also factors. Scientific evidence
links endometriosis with a weakened immune system as
well. There's no cure.

Conventional treatment calls for hormone therapy
medications, which suppress estrogen and lessen uncomfortable symptoms. In some cases, women have hysterec-
tomies. You may be able to avoid these drastic measures by
finding herbal treatments that alleviate most symptoms.
After speaking with your natural health care professional,
select herbs that reduce bleeding, swelling, muscle aches,
cramping, and pain.

Ease pain with a nourishing tea. To fend off intense
pain, herbalists often recommend this relaxing, nourishing
tea as the first step in a natural treatment plan for endometriosis. Combine equal parts of passionflower,
skullcap, and damiana. Passionflower and skullcap ease
pain; damiana relieves stress. Then add equal parts of alfalfa leaf, nettle, and raspberry leaf (which also balances
hormones). All three of these herbs have a long history of
relieving menstrual problems. For tea, steep 1 tablespoon
of this blend in 8 ounces of freshly boiled water for at least

1 hour in a covered container. Strain and sip. Have up to 3 cups of the tea a day.

Sip your way to improvement. For a front-line assault against the most intense symptoms of endometriosis, try this multi-herb blend tea that herbalists say balances hormones, curbs excessive bleeding, stops body-bending pain, and reduces inflammation.

Combine 1 teaspoon each of dried chasteberry, echinacea root, wild yam, and cramp bark with ½ teaspoon each of dried horsetail, raspberry leaf, and motherwort. Place these herbs in an uncovered pan with 1 quart of cold water and bring to a boil. Turn down the heat and simmer for 5 minutes. Remove from the heat, cover, and steep for 15 minutes. Strain out the herbs and drink 2 cups daily.

Make cramps disappear with a four-herb formula. For excruciating cramps, try a combination of Jamaican dogwood, kava kava, white willow bark, and valerian. Herbalists recommend taking 10 drops of each herb, in undiluted tincture form, 2 hours before bedtime and again right before you go to sleep. These herbs provide pain relief, stop muscle aches and spasms, and ease nervous tension.

If you try this tincture formula, don't exceed the recommended dose, and use it only as needed, not on an ongoing basis. Since it can make you drowsy, use it only before bed or when you'll be home all day. Do not use it when you'll be driving.

Fatigue

Okay, so you're not the Energizer Bunny. Who is? In the real world, meeting the demands of job, family, home, and community leaves many of us exhausted. Instead of *going, going, going*, we wish we could just go to bed.

Many people say they're tapped out from trying to do

too much in too little time. Their fatigue comes not just from feeling overextended but also from feeling stressed. In response, they find themselves reaching for quick pick-me-ups—another cup of coffee, another piece of chocolate, another snack cake from the vending machine. The trouble is that stimulants like caffeine and sugar may eventually leave them feeling even more exhausted.

The alternative? First, get a handle on why you're feeling so tired—and rule out underlying medical conditions. Ask yourself: How long have I been tired? Have I been under stress for a long time? What's making me so exhausted and why? Then take that information to your doctor.

If the checkup rules out medical conditions and determines that you're basically healthy, consider recharging with these herbal fatigue-blasting strategies.

Inhale peppermint for a quick lift. Rather than reaching for the coffeepot when you need a quick pick-me-up, grab a bottle of peppermint essential oil and inhale its stimulating scent. You can also put peppermint oil in a diffuser, a pump that blows the scent into the air. Place the diffuser in a convenient location, such as on your desk at work or on the end table in your living room. Or you can just sprinkle a few drops of the essential oil into a small bowl of hot water. The steam will waft the scent through the air.

Grab Siberian ginseng for stamina. Siberian ginseng increases your resistance to all kinds of stress. Place 1 teaspoon of dried Siberian ginseng in a cup of boiling water, steep, strain, and then drink. It will take up to a month of continuous use before you'll notice any effects from using ginseng.

Be better with basil. Relieve mental fatigue with spicy basil essential oil. Add some droplets to a diffuser or sprinkle on a handkerchief and sniff when you feel tired.

Fever

To a certain extent, fever is your body's ally. When a virus or bacterium invades your body, your immune system literally turns up the heat to melt away infection or inflammation. This biological furnace enhances your body's ability to fend off these intruders.

Keeping that in mind, natural healers say you should let a fever run its course so that it can destroy infectious organisms and help you get well. If you suppress a fever too quickly, you hinder your immune system's attempt to defeat the invader. But if a fever goes above 103°F or lasts more than 24 hours, call your doctor. And if you do let a fever run its course, remember to drink plenty of fluids—otherwise, you may risk dehydration.

While over-the-counter medications may take the edge off a fever, herbal treatments promote sweating so that it can run its course more quickly and effectively. Taking herbs may actually make you feel temporarily more feverish, but be patient. In the end, you'll likely feel a lot better.

Break a fever fast, with yarrow and more. To work up a sweat and break a fever, try this three-herb tea. Combine equal parts of dried elderflower, yarrow, and peppermint. Place 4½ teaspoons of this mix in a pint canning jar. Boil 2 cups of water and pour it into the jar over the herbs. Cover and let it steep for 3 to 4 hours. Strain and add honey to taste. This recipe makes 2 cups. After drinking a cup or two of this tea, you will start to sweat. Once that happens, you have had enough. Check with your naturopathic physician if you are unable to find some of these herbs.

> **• Herb at a Glance •**
> **Ginseng.** Good for stress, fatigue, and memory loss as well as protecting the liver

Take nature's aspirin. For high fevers that cause body aches, turn to nature's original aspirin, willow bark. This herb contains salicin, the active ingredient in aspirin that reduces pain and swelling. For best results, swallow three or four 200-milligram capsules of willow bark extract a day while you have a fever. Make sure to buy a standardized formula that contains 15 percent salicin.

Replenish with natural ginger ale. If you're dehydrated, fresh, natural ginger ale will restore needed fluids and fight the germs that caused your fever. Try this easy-to-make natural ginger ale tea: In a saucepan, combine 1 teaspoon of thinly sliced fresh ginger (or ½ teaspoon ginger powder), 1 teaspoon of raspberry leaves, and 3 cups of water. Bring to a boil. Turn down the heat and simmer for 5 minutes. Remove from the heat and steep for 10 minutes. Strain out the herbs. Add 1 cup of carbonated water and one lemon slice just before you're ready to drink.

Gas

Most times, flatulence is nothing more than an annoyance. But sometimes, the sheer volume of gas in the intestines causes bloating, discomfort, and pain. Most of the gas you pass forms when undigested food wends its way into your large intestine and gets broken down by bacteria that live there.

Gender doesn't play a role. Eating habits, however, can be important. People who eat more protein than vegetables tend to have more flatulence because protein is a major source of sulfur, a gassy compound. Those people with lactose intolerance, a condition in which they have trouble digesting milk sugar (lactose), also experience more gas. The artificial sweetener sorbitol triggers gas as well.

Although it's impossible to be flatulence-free, these

herbs can help you control the intensity and frequency of untimely outbursts.

Put on the brakes with fennel. To ensure you're free of excess gas, chew ½ teaspoon of fennel seeds. Fennel is a carminative, a substance that helps dissipate gas. It also helps correct digestive disturbances by relaxing muscle spasms.

Run out of gas with peppermint. Peppermint, another carminative, is a digestive soother with a reputation for minimizing gas. For best results, pour 1 cup of just-boiled water over 1 tablespoon of dried peppermint leaves. Steep, covered, for 5 to 10 minutes, then strain and sip. Drink a cup of this tea three or four times daily.

Caution: Avoid drinking this tea if you have esophageal reflux.

Season with gas-banishing spices. If you enjoy eating beans or other gas-producing foods, you can tone down the tooting by seasoning your dishes with herbs from the mint and carrot families, herbalists suggest. Keep eating beans, which are an excellent source of high-quality protein, fiber, and other nutrients, but also reach for aniseed, basil, chamomile, cinnamon, garlic, ginger, lemon, onion, oregano, or rosemary—all of which are excellent carminatives.

Gum Problems

Plaque turns white teeth a dirty shade of yellow, but this sticky film does its worst damage where you can't see it: below the gum line. In fact, plaque ranks as the top cause of gum disease, taking responsibility for about 80 percent of all dental problems in adults.

If you don't brush and floss daily, plaque—a soft, bacteria-packed film that forms on and between your teeth and under your gum line—becomes a rock-hard substance called tartar. Tartar irritates gums, causing them to swell,

---

• *Herb at a Glance* •

Goldenseal. Good for sinus infections, colds and flu, laryngitis, sore throats, earaches, gastritis, and colitis

---

bleed, and become infected. These symptoms are signs of gingivitis, an early stage of gum disease.

Pregnant women are especially prone to gingivitis, especially during the first trimester. The rise in risk is related to rising levels of the female hormone estrogen during pregnancy, which seem to encourage certain types of plaque-forming bacteria to grow.

If you ignore gingivitis, your condition can worsen into periodontitis, causing gums to severely recede and teeth to loosen from your jawbone. But gum disease need not progress that far. Practicing mouth maintenance—brushing and flossing thoroughly and getting regular dental exams—will significantly safeguard the health of your gums.

You can also try these herbal treatments for additional gum-health insurance.

Herbalize your tooth brushing. In addition to your regular brushing and flossing routine, heal inflamed, diseased gums with goldenseal. Mix 1 tablespoon of goldenseal powder with enough water to form a paste. Then brush your teeth as you normally would. This bitter-tasting herb contains two alkaloids, hydrastine and berberine, that are potent antibiotics and inflammation fighters.

Fortify your water jet with echinacea. Fight off plaque and bacteria caused by food particles lodged in your teeth with a dental hygiene device (such as a Water Pik) that uses a high-speed water jet. Then bolster its healing powers by adding 2 to 4 drops of echinacea tincture to its water reservoir. Echinacea is acclaimed by herbalists as an effective oral antibacterial agent.

Drink chamomile after meals. If your gums are swollen and infected, drink a cup of chamomile tea after every meal. This herb helps to stop inflammation and kill germs, and it helps prevent gum disease. Infuse 2 teaspoons of dried chamomile in a cup of just-boiled water. Then let it steep for 5 to 10 minutes before drinking.

Sip or chew peppermint. Peppermint leaves help prevent gum disease by fighting the bacteria that cause tooth decay. To make a tea, steep 2 teaspoons of crushed fresh peppermint leaves in a cup of just-boiled water for 10 minutes. Then strain and sip. Or you can chew fresh mint leaves.

Hay Fever

Chalk up all that wheezing and sneezing to annoying airborne pollen. Hay fever occurs when your immune system goes a little haywire. Instead of limiting its assaults to bacteria and viruses, it attacks harmless stuff like pollen, flooding your body with defensive chemicals called histamines. Unfortunately, this all-out response causes congestion, a runny nose, and itchy, watery eyes.

Some people find that pollen from flowering plants brings on hay fever's worst symptoms every year. You can enjoy the changing seasons by turning to nature's best hay fever fighters.

Breathe relief with nettle. Prepare yourself for the approaching hay fever season by drinking nettle tea for at least 1 month ahead of time. This herb contains trace amounts of histamines, which stimulate your body to build immunity through its own natural antihistamine. To make nettle tea, pour 1 cup of boiling water over 1 to 3 teaspoons of dried nettle. Steep for 10 to 15 minutes, then strain. Drink 3 cups a day. For best results, continue sipping the tea regularly during allergy season and for 1 month after it ends.

Make an herbal blend. For relief from sneezing and congestion and to bolster your immune system, combine ½ teaspoon each of tinctures of Siberian ginseng, nettle, elderflowers, and peppermint. Take half a dropperful at least five times daily, starting a few weeks before hay fever season begins. Siberian ginseng boosts immunity, and elderflowers help stop sneezing and relieve congestion. Peppermint helps clear congestion.

Headaches

Muscle contractions characterize tension headaches, the most common type of head pain. Pain usually starts in the muscles at the back of your head and neck, then it works its way to your forehead. Or you may simply feel a mild, steady throbbing just behind your eyes or in your temples. Stress is often the trigger, but marathon, eye-straining stints at your computer or sitting in a cramped position for a long time can also cause a tension headache.

Fortunately, these headaches usually disappear within a few hours, or even faster when you take aspirin or another over-the-counter pain reliever. But if aspirin isn't working or if you're worried about its side effects, then consider these safe herbal alternatives to quiet the throbbing and relax the tension that brought on pain in the first place.

Tame pain with feverfew or cramp bark. To stop the dull ache of a tension headache, take feverfew or cramp bark every hour for up to 3 hours. Follow the label directions on the tincture or capsule bottles for the proper dosage. Feverfew contains salicylic acid, the active ingredient in aspirin, but in lower concentrations. Cramp bark has antispasmodic properties that herbalists say help relax tight muscles.

Reach for "herbal aspirin." For a pounding headache, try white willow, often nicknamed herbal aspirin. White willow contains salicin, an aspirin-like chemical that is easily absorbed by your digestive tract. Unlike aspirin, however, willow bark probably won't irritate your stomach.

Soak away the pain with lemon balm and lavender. If your head throbs at night, a lukewarm herbal bath may bring relief. Add 2 tablespoons of dried lemon balm and 2 tablespoons of lavender flowers to a cup of just-boiled water. Steep 10 minutes, then strain. Pour this tea into a tub filled with lukewarm water. Ease in and soak for 20 minutes. Lavender and lemon balm are both known as relaxing herbs.

Mellow the ache with a calming herbal tea. For simple tension headaches, select one or more of these relaxing herbs: chamomile, linden flower, lemon balm, or passionflower. Brew a cup of tea using 1 teaspoon of your chosen dried herb or herb blend per cup of just-boiled water. Steep 5 to 10 minutes, strain, and sip. Between sips, take deep, relaxing breaths as your headache disappears.

Heartburn

Maybe your heart isn't really on fire—but something inside you sure feels incendiary. That feeling comes from the sizzle that happens whenever stomach acid trespasses into the esophagus, the sensitive tube that connects your mouth to your stomach.

Heartburn usually strikes about an hour after a big meal or after you've eaten sugary or high-fat foods. That's because the cardiac sphincter, a gatekeeping muscle between your esophagus and stomach, gives way to pressure when you've eaten more than your body can handle. The muscle ring weakens and opens, allowing corrosive stomach acid to reflux, that is, to backflow and irritate the esophagus.

Many people rely on over-the-counter antacids to cool heartburn, but prolonged use of antacids can actually worsen esophageal problems over time. If your heartburn

THE HERBAL KITCHEN

Stop Heartburn with Dill Tea

For more than 3,000 years, many cultures have turned to dill to ease digestive pain. In fact, the word *dill* comes from the Old Norse word *dilla*, meaning "to lull or soothe." A cup of this dill tea, recommended by Shez Ward, an herbalist in Norfolk, England, and a member of the Royal Horticultural Society, will keep calm a stomach bothered by heartburn and indigestion.

3 teaspoons dill seeds
1 cup boiling water
Honey (to taste)

Using a spoon, bruise or pound the dill seeds until they break into small pieces. Put the seeds in a pot and cover them with the water. Put the lid on and let the tea steep for 30 minutes. Strain the tea and add honey to taste.

is occurring three or four times a week for weeks on end, it's time to see a doctor. Heartburn may be a symptom of something more serious. But if you have garden-variety heartburn, your doctor may tell you to continue taking antacids. What can you do instead? Herbalists advise that you stay clear of fatty or sugary foods, cut back on coffee, and drink plenty of water. Then try these herbal strategies.

Banish the burn with licorice. If you're prone to heartburn, take licorice before each meal. Deglycyrrhizinated licorice reduces the frequency of flare-ups by encouraging cells that line your stomach to produce mucus, which provides a "safety coating" that protects against your own highly acidic digestive juices. Take two 500-milligram tablets of deglycyrrhizinated licorice root 15 minutes before meals for best results. Make sure that you choose deglycyrrhizinated licorice, because it does not contain glycyrrhizin, a substance that can raise blood pressure.

Activate your digestion with turmeric. Season food with turmeric to keep your digestive juices flowing smoothly and food moving through your gastrointestinal tract without a hitch. If seasoning your food isn't enough to stop heartburn, take two or three turmeric capsules (for a total of ½ to 1 gram) before each meal.

Cool the fire with chamomile. Subdue heartburn pain, or prevent a new attack, with chamomile—a mild sedative that soothes mucous membranes. To make chamomile tea, add 1 tablespoon of whole dried chamomile flowers to 1 cup of hot water and steep for 15 minutes. Strain and drink daily. Some herbalists recommend that you keep the teapot and your cup covered so that the vapor can't escape. The volatile oils in the vapor are among chamomile's active ingredients.

Hemorrhoids

In and around your anus and rectum are tiny, hardworking veins that expand during a bowel movement and shrink back to shape afterward. If you overtax them from prolonged sitting, straining while you're constipated, or lifting heavy objects, these veins surrender to pressure and can swell, ache, itch—or leave a harmless dab of blood on toilet paper after a bowel movement.

Happily, most hemorrhoids come and go on their own within a few days. You can discourage these uncomfortable swellings by eating plenty of high-fiber foods and drinking lots of fluids. This combination of fiber and fluids helps bulk up the stool so it becomes softer and passes more easily through the rectum and anus.

Beyond these dietary tips, herbalists offer the following soothing botanical remedies for hemorrhoids.

Stop pain and swelling with witch hazel. If you experience painful, inflamed hemorrhoids, soak in a witch hazel sitz bath. Pour a pint of witch hazel into a tub filled with a couple inches of warm water. Sit in it for at least 15 minutes. Witch hazel acts as an astringent that shrinks swollen tissues and soothes pain.

Get your bowels moving with psyllium. For hemorrhoids brought on by the pushing and straining of constipation, turn to psyllium seed husks. Take 4 to 10 teaspoons of psyllium per day until symptoms vanish. Psyllium is a form of fiber that swells as it absorbs water in the stomach, adding bulk to stool and triggering muscle contractions that speed the waste along.

Soften stools with butternut. To soften stools and ease pain, herbalists suggest taking 20 to 30 drops of butternut tincture three times a day until your hemorrhoids disappear.

Herpes

An alarming number of people have one of the two forms of *Herpes simplex*, the virus that leaves clusters of fluid-filled blisters around the mouth or the genitals. Only half of those people exposed to the virus experience any symptoms, yet even symptom-free herpes carriers can be contagious—and can unintentionally spread the virus to others.

If you do come in contact with herpes, the first symptoms can surface within 7 days of contact. Your mouth or genitals—or both—may tingle, burn, and itch. Then blisters appear, your skin reddens, and finally, the painful blisters burst. After that, herpes goes back into hiding until the next outbreak.

Like the common cold, herpes has yet to be conquered and cured, though antiviral medications may lessen the severity of an outbreak and increase the time between outbreaks. If you feel a burning or tingling in your genital area, followed by the eruption of small, red blisters that form a shallow ulcer, see your doctor. It goes without saying that you should nix sex if you or your partner has herpes blisters. While you can't stop this surly virus, you can subdue its symptoms and keep it dormant for as long as possible with these herbal strategies.

Bag herpes with black tea. To reduce pain and inflammation during a herpes attack, steep a tea bag filled with black tea for a few minutes in just enough boiling water to cover it. Let the bag cool and apply it directly to the herpes lesion. Black tea contains astringent tannins that may help dry out an outbreak.

Rely on lemon balm. Fight herpes with lemon balm, which contains compounds called polyphenols that prevent the virus from attaching to your body's cells, thus preventing the spread of infection.

Make a strong tea by steeping 2 to 4 teaspoons of dried lemon balm in a cup of just-boiled water. Strain, then let the tea cool. Apply it directly to herpes blisters with a cotton ball several times a day.

Make a minty anti-herpes tea. Combine the virus-fighting power of lemon balm and other mint-family herbs in a tea that herbal experts say contains a dozen anti-herpes compounds. Fill a saucepan halfway with water and bring to a boil. Turn off the heat and add fresh lemon balm leaves

> • *Herb at a Glance* •
> **Lavender.** Good for headaches, muscle spasms and cramps, depression, and digestive upsets

until the pan is about three-quarters full. (If fresh lemon balm is not available, substitute ¼ cup of dried lemon balm.) Then add two parts each of dried oregano and self-heal and one part each of hyssop, rosemary, sage, and thyme. (The exact amounts don't matter as long as there's twice as much oregano and self-heal.) Toss in a little licorice root as a sweetener and steep the mixture for 20 minutes before straining and drinking.

Keep the virus at bay with burdock and echinacea. To prevent recurrent outbreaks of herpes, create a gentle tonic, using burdock root and echinacea. Prepare a very strong tea by using 1 ounce of each herb to 1 quart of water. Toss the dried herbs into a quart jar and fill it to the top with boiling water. Steep for 4 to 8 hours, then strain. Drink ½ cup two to four times a day to limit outbreaks. Burdock acts as a mild antiviral agent and echinacea stimulates the immune system. Stop taking this infusion if you go 3 months with no outbreaks.

High Blood Pressure

High blood pressure occurs when circulating blood exerts too much pressure on artery walls, causing scarring, thickening, and hardening. Not only are arteries damaged, but your heart must pump harder to get the blood through. Stress, inactivity, a diet high in fats, and obesity all raise your risk for high blood pressure. Undetected and untreated, it can lead to two of America's top killers: heart disease and stroke.

Only a blood pressure test can tell you whether or not your blood pressure is within safe ranges. For adults, a blood pressure reading of 120/80 mm Hg (millimeters of mercury) is considered normal; a consistent reading of 140/90 mm Hg is considered high. Doctors recommend annual blood pressure screenings to be sure that your pressure stays within the safe ranges.

Fortunately, eating more fresh fruits and vegetables and getting regular physical exercise can help control or prevent runaway blood pressure. So can incorporating these herbal remedies into your life.

Jazz up your food with garlic. To lower blood pressure as well as cholesterol, natural healers suggest eating a clove of garlic daily. Studies have shown that a compound in garlic called allicin successfully deflates high blood pressure. Simply cook with garlic and use it in your salads. If you don't like its taste, take garlic in capsule form, following the label directions.

Take lemon balm for relief. For high blood pressure triggered by stress, try a daily dose of lemon balm. Take 5 milliliters of lemon balm tincture twice a day for 12 weeks. Then recheck your blood pressure and continue taking as needed. Herbalists say lemon balm calms as it lifts your spirits, which can translate into lower blood pressure readings.

Help your heart with hawthorn. To help strengthen your heart, reach for hawthorn, a centuries-old heart tonic. Make a tea using 1 teaspoon of dried hawthorn per cup of boiling water and drink 2 cups per day. Or you can take 5 milliliters of hawthorn tincture twice a day. Hawthorn widens blood vessels, especially the coronary arteries, thereby lowering blood pressure.

High Cholesterol

You've no doubt heard that too much cholesterol in your blood—or in your diet—can contribute to heart disease. But did you know that cholesterol isn't all bad? Your body needs some in order to function properly.

In fact, your body produces its own cholesterol to make

adrenal and sex hormones. In addition, you need the good-guy, high-density lipoprotein (HDL) cholesterol around in order to help boot out the bad-guy, low-density lipoprotein (LDL) cholesterol, which clogs arteries.

Medical experts have set healthy levels for cholesterol at 60 milligrams per deciliter of blood for HDL and 130 milligrams per deciliter or less for LDL. Levels of LDLs above 130 heighten your risk for arteriosclerosis, a condition in which fatty deposits build up on the walls of your arteries. Blocked arteries lead to heart attacks and strokes.

Fortunately, you can lower your cholesterol with a low-fat diet and exercise. Beyond that, try these herbal helpers.

Go heavy on garlic. For a proven cholesterol reducer that also lowers blood pressure, get garlic. Eat three to

A Natural Solution to a Cholesterol Problem

Although she's under 40, Geraldine has had high levels of cholesterol and triglycerides for years. If she can't get them under control, her risk for heart disease will escalate. She has read that an herb known as guggul can lower both triglycerides and cholesterol. She wants to give it a try, but her doctor may not be enthusiastic about her using an herb he has never heard of instead of medications he knows.

What can Geraldine do to help her case? First, she needs to educate herself as well as her doctor about this herb. A little research would reveal that guggul has been used in India for thousands of years, and its uses worldwide have ranged from treating arthritis to lowering high cholesterol, notes Nancy Lonsdorf, M.D., an Ayurvedic practitioner and medical director of the Maharishi Vedic four fresh cloves a day in foods (minced and added to salads, soups, sauces, and stews) or take garlic capsules containing 3,000 to 4,000 micrograms of allicin (one of the active compounds in garlic) daily. More than 30 years of research shows that garlic lowers cholesterol and reduces heart disease risk. Some research suggests garlic also prevents the formation of blood clots that can block arteries.

Grab some guggul. Guggul is a gum resin closely related to myrrh. Some natural healers say it can raise HDL levels by as much as 20 percent and lower LDL levels by the same percentage.

Guggul creates more LDL receptors in the liver. They take more of the bad cholesterol out of your blood and ex-

Medical Center in Rockville, Maryland. In fact, 80 percent of people who took guggul in one study lowered their cholesterol by 24 percent and their triglycerides by 23 percent.

More and more doctors are open to recommending herbal remedies now that there is so much public interest in alternative medicine. If Geraldine's doctor isn't, she should find out why. He may have a good reason for his point of view. If she still feels strongly about giving herbs a shot, maybe she should look for a doctor who is less close-minded.

Whatever Geraldine decides, she should continue to have her cholesterol levels checked every 3 months. And she should avoid guggul if she has an ulcer, heavy menstrual flow, or problems with acid reflux—a cause of heartburn. Guggul can aggravate these conditions.

crete it through the feces before it can make fat deposits in your arteries.

Look for guggul products in standardized form. The recommended standardized dose is 25 milligrams three times a day. Take guggul until your lipid levels have normalized, and then reduce the dose to 25 milligrams once a day.

Sow health with fenugreek seed. Cut your LDL levels by consuming 1 to 2 tablespoons of ground fenugreek seeds three or four times a day. Fenugreek, which has a bittersweet taste, is best sprinkled on food or sipped as an herbal tea. Steep 1 teaspoon of ground seed in one cup of freshly boiled water. If you don't like its taste, take one or two 580-milligram capsules of fenugreek three or four times a day for the same LDL-lowering results.

Hot Flashes

In no time flat, a hot flash can work you into a sweat. In just a matter of seconds, the sensation of sweat and heat drenches your face, neck, chest, and sometimes your entire body. Shivering chills follow as your body reacts to wide-open pores and soaked skin.

Of all the changes heralding menopause, most women rate these heated surges as the most notorious. Three out of every four American women experience them during the transition from monthly periods to menopause. They can occur at any time during the day or night.

No one knows exactly what provokes hot flashes, but some experts suggest that hormonal changes may irritate blood vessels and nerves, causing the blood vessels to overdilate. Others theorize that a hot flash kicks in when levels of the female hormone estrogen plummet.

Estrogen influences the hypothalamus, your brain's thermostat. When estrogen levels drop, your body's ability to regulate your temperature goes haywire. Blood surges to the surface of your skin. Your skin temperature rises a little, and your heartbeat and breathing speed up slightly. As your body desperately tries to cool itself, you perspire. Because the hot flash dissipates heat, your body's core temperature drops, making you feel cold and clammy. Total time elapsed: just 2 to 5 minutes.

Fortunately, hot flashes are physically harmless, but they can make you feel flustered and self-conscious—or leave you feeling irritable and fatigued if they strike while you sleep. The first few may take you by surprise, but eventually you'll learn to anticipate their arrival. When a hot flash is on the way, reach for one of these herbal remedies.

Tame the flash with motherwort and more. To moderate hot flashes day or night, turn to motherwort and black cohosh. Mix two parts of motherwort tincture with one part black cohosh tincture. Take ¼ teaspoon of this formula, mixed into a little water or a cup of tea, three times per day. Motherwort has been scientifically proven to strengthen your heart by lowering blood pressure, which may be why it reduces hot flashes. It also has sedative qualities to fight insomnia. Black cohosh contains estrogen-like substances that relieve the discomforts of hot flashes.

Cool down fast with chickweed. To reduce the severity and frequency of hot flashes, herbalists recommend taking 25 to 40 drops of chickweed tincture once or twice a day. Most women see improvement within a week or two of regular use.

Indigestion

It could have been those three helpings of pecan pie last night or the way you gulped down breakfast in the car on your way to work this morning. Maybe it was just stress. Whatever the cause, your stomach is burning, and you feel gassy and bloated—and way too full.

THE HERBAL KITCHEN

Natural Ginger Ale for Stomach Upset

To soothe an upset stomach, make your own ginger ale, as recommended by herbalist Kathi Keville, director of the American Herb Association and author of *Herbs for Health and Healing*.

- 1 teaspoon finely chopped fresh ginger or ½ teaspoon powdered ginger
- 1 teaspoon red raspberry leaves
- 3 cups water
- 1 cup carbonated water
- 1 lemon slice

Place the ginger, raspberry leaves, and plain water in a saucepan. Bring to a boil, then reduce the heat and simmer for 5 minutes. Remove from heat and steep for 10 minutes. Strain out the herbs. Add the carbonated water and lemon just before serving. Drink as much as you desire.

Simply stated, you have indigestion. Here's what to do.

Ease the ache with peppermint. To calm your stomach and dispel gas, try a cup of peppermint tea. You will get the best results by growing your own peppermint and using the fresh or dried leaves. But store-bought peppermint tea can also help. Use 1 tablespoon of whole dried leaves (2 tablespoons of fresh leaves) or one tea bag per cup of hot water. Steep for 10 minutes. Sip slowly, allowing yourself—and your stomach—to relax. If indigestion is common, have a cup in the morning and one at night to prevent it.

Speed digestion with ginger. Soothe your stomach and aid digestion with ginger tea. Steep 1 teaspoon of grated fresh ginger in a cup of just-boiled water. Strain and sip. Ginger contains gingerols and shogaols, chemicals that stimulate the wavelike muscle contractions (known as peristalsis) that move food from the stomach to the small intestine.

Sip an herbal aperitif. To stop indigestion before it starts, quaff this five-herb aperitif about 30 minutes before meals. Herbalists say this drink primes your digestive system for your meal and helps it more easily break down the food into nutrients.

Combine 1 ounce dried gentian root (ground and sifted), ½ ounce dried barberry (ground and sifted), ½ ounce dried angelica (ground and sifted), ¼ ounce crushed dried fennel seeds, and ¼ ounce crushed dried cardamom seeds in a glass container with a tight lid. When you're not using them, store in a cool location. Before a big meal, add 1 teaspoon of the herb mix to one cup of boiling water. Cover and simmer for 15 minutes. Allow the tea to cool, then strain. Have ½ cup 30 minutes before a meal. (You can refrigerate the other ½ cup, covered, to use the next day.) Drink this aperitif tea warm or cold, but don't add ice. Ice will suppress digestion and hamper these herbs from doing their job. Dried gentian root and dried angelica may be difficult to find, so check with your naturopathic physician.

Finish with fennel. At the close of a big meal, ward off indigestion by chewing a teaspoon of fennel seeds. The naturally bitter taste gets your digestive juices flowing. It's a traditional choice in India and is often offered after meals at Indian restaurants in the United States.

Infertility

Long before the emergence of fertility drugs, ovulation test kits, sperm analysis, and infertility clinics, plant remedies were used as a means of reversing infertility.

Many fertility herbs used today come to us from ancient Chinese and Native American herbal medicine traditions. Experts in alternative medicine recommend matching good nutrition, exercise, and stress reduction with herbs to enhance fertility.

If you want to reverse infertility, you'll have to figure out what's causing it. Work with your doctor to determine what's going on in your particular case. Surgery or drug treatments may be needed. Or you may find that herbal remedies can help balance hormone levels and restore overall vitality. Here's how.

Sip a six-herb formula. To enhance fertility, drink 2 cups of this fertility tea daily: In a pot, combine 1 teaspoon each of dried dong quai (also known as dang gui), Siberian ginseng, and chasteberry (also known as vitex) with 1 teaspoon each of dried motherwort leaves, cramp bark, and wild yam in 1 quart of water. Simmer for 5 minutes. Turn off the heat and steep for 20 minutes. Strain out the herbs before drinking.

Dong quai and cramp bark relax the uterus and help regulate menstrual irregularities. Siberian ginseng fights stress. Chasteberry helps balance hormones. Motherwort is used for a variety of female conditions, and wild yam is reputed to have estrogenic effects.

Over 40? Start with dandelion. If you're over 40 and want to have a baby, herbalists often recommend you start to revitalize your body by taking bitters like dandelion root before meals. Try 5 to 10 drops of dandelion root tincture right before you eat. Add bitter "gourmet" greens, such as dandelion leaves and arugula, to your salads, too. Since your body slows down the production of enzymes as you age, you may need to boost your body's ability to absorb nutrients before trying fertility-enhancing herbs. Research shows dandelion contains bitter compounds that stimulate the secretion of bile, which aids in digestion.

Insomnia

Coast to coast, as many as 50 million Americans regularly miss out on a good night's rest. Some take a long time to doze off. Others wake up from sleep repeatedly during the night. Still others fall into dreamland quickly, only to wake at 2:00 A.M. and find themselves unable to fall back to sleep.

Sleepless nights usually turn into sleepy days. Many people need between 8 and 8½ hours of sleep each night. Losing even an hour or so each night can rob you of your normal get-up-and-go. You may lack energy, drive, and concentration or find that you become irritated more easily.

Lifestyle adjustments, such as avoiding coffee at night and exercising a few times a week, can help fight insomnia. So can meditation and progressive relaxation techniques. Natural healers also suggest these herbs for a good night's sleep.

Cap the night with lemon balm. For a safe sedative that also soothes your stomach, herbalists suggest a cup of lemon balm tea at bedtime. Use 1 to 3 teaspoons of the dried herb per cup of just-boiled water. Cover, steep for 10 minutes, and strain. Chemicals in the plant, called terpenes, help provide a sedative action.

Find slumber with valerian. If you're looking for an herbal alternative to tranquilizers, select valerian. The herb's active ingredient includes a group of compounds called valepotriates. Research shows that these compounds attach to the same brain receptors as tranquilizers. Valerian is not one of the best tasting or smelling herbs, so herbalists recom-

---

• *Herb at a Glance* •

Lemon balm. Good for relieving depression, insomnia, nervousness, tension headaches, and digestive problems related to stress

mend you take one or two 400-milligram capsules (rather than tea or tincture) about 30 minutes before bed for best results.

Begin the morning with a relaxing herb. Don't wait until bedtime to take herbs that soothe the nervous system

Make an Herbal Sleep Pillow

Since the dawn of time, people have relied on herb-filled pillows to lull them to sleep. Tucked away inside a small sack, herbs believed to heal the nervous system chased away restlessness and insomnia, says herbalist Rosemary Gladstar, director of the Sage Mountain Herbal Education Center in East Barre, Vermont.

To make a sleep pillow, fold a piece of 8-inch-by-8-inch fabric in half (with right sides facing). Soft fabrics such as cotton, flannel, and velvet are best. If you like, embroider or decorate the fabric first. Sew two of the sides together, leaving one side open for stuffing. Turn the fabric right side out.

In a bowl, mix together one part lavender, one part hops, one part chamomile, and one part rose. (Hops can occasionally cause a skin rash, so handle fresh or dried hops carefully.) Stuff the mixture into the fabric. Six to 8 ounces of the herb mixture should be enough to fill the pillow. Sew closed the remaining open side.

Place the herbal pillow beside your head or inside your regular pillow at night. Fluff it before you go to sleep to release the odors. The pillow will last for several years, but if you like, you can renew the herbs every year.

To make a dream pillow to stimulate your dreams, simply add mugwort to the herb mixture. It's an herb that herbalists believe really gets you dreaming.

and promote restful sleep. By keeping calm all day, you'll find it much easier to slip into dreamland after dark. Choose either passionflower, skullcap, or St. John's wort. Use 1 tablespoon of dried herb per cup of just-boiled water. Steep for an hour, strain, and sip.

Jet Lag

Whether you're traveling for business or pleasure, jet lag can leave you feeling foggy headed and physically sapped.

When you fly across several time zones, it takes time for your internal body clock to adjust to the new local day/night cycle. Until it resets itself, you may feel irritable and experience headaches, fatigue, an upset stomach, or insomnia. Traveling from east to west—say, from New York to Honolulu—is easier on your internal clock than journeying west to east. That's because you're pushing your body clock backward instead of forward. Sleep disorder specialists say that it's easier to stay up later—and wake up later—than to try to go to sleep earlier and get up earlier.

On its own, your body needs about 1 day of adjustment for every time zone you cross. But if you're taking a short vacation, you might not be fully adjusted until it's time to board the plane home. You can gently encourage your internal clock to reset more quickly and help yourself adjust more comfortably to your new surroundings with these herbal travel helpers.

Adapt with ginseng. Aid your adjustment to new surroundings in a different time zone by taking 250 milligrams of Siberian ginseng in capsule form twice daily. Start taking Siberian ginseng 4 days before a long flight, then take it during the flight and for 4 days after you arrive at your destination. This herb will help overcome the stress of adapting to a new time zone.

Tuck fragrant herbs in your pillow. For peaceful sleep upon arrival, dab a drop each of the essential oils of ylang-ylang, lavender, and frankincense on a tissue, suggest herbal experts. Tuck the tissue under your pillow and get some well-deserved Zzzs. Ylang-ylang wards off depression and nervous tension; lavender eases insomnia; and frankincense is believed to soothe the spirit. Women who find that traveling disrupts their menstrual cycles or makes PMS worse should add a drop of rose geranium to the formula. This herb helps normalize hormones.

Arrive alert with essential oils. If you need to be sharp and alert as soon as you step off of the plane, aromatherapy experts suggest you pack these energizing essential oils: rosemary, basil, eucalyptus, and peppermint. Dab a drop of each on a tissue or handkerchief. Breathe in every time your eyelids start to close. Rosemary stimulates your nervous system, basil overcomes mental fatigue, eucalyptus is an energy booster, and peppermint counters mental fogginess.

Pack herbal tea bags. In addition to your suitcases, don't forget to pack chamomile tea bags. Dunk the tea bags in cool water and place them on the skin just below your eyes to combat fatigue-induced puffiness. Drink a cup of chamomile tea once you arrive, to help you relax after a long and stressful trip.

Laryngitis

The mouth opens, the lips and tongue form words, but the voice . . . where's the voice? Don't panic. It's only laryngitis.

Similar to a sore throat, laryngitis dries out the mucous membranes that surround the larynx, or voice box. When this membrane can't moisten or filter air properly, your speaking voice, which is created by air passing over your vocal cords, becomes whispery or totally disappears. A cold or flu, excessive shouting, or even singing can cause voice loss.

Fortunately, herbal healers say you can regain your voice with herbs.

Say it with herbal steam. When a virus or excessive talking robs you of your voice, heal your larynx and vocal cords naturally with an essential-oil steam. Bring 3 cups of water to a simmer and turn off the heat. Add ¼ teaspoon of eucalyptus or peppermint essential oil. Place the pot in front of you. Position your face over the pot at a distance so that the steam doesn't burn your face, and drape a towel over the back of your head to form a mini-sauna. Breathe in the steam for 10 to 15 minutes, coming out for fresh air as needed.

Do this at least three times a day. Eucalyptus contains a chemical called cineole that researchers believe may relieve sore throat inflammation and fight infection. Peppermint contains substances believed to kill many kinds of microorganisms.

Lose laryngitis with a spicy juice. For laryngitis induced by a cold, herbalists recommend this mixture of lemon, honey, and ground red pepper. Squeeze the juice from one to two fresh lemons, then mix the juice with a tablespoon of honey and a pinch of ground red pepper. Take a small sip of the mixture every few hours throughout the day. Ground red pepper (also known as cayenne pepper) thins phlegm and eases its passage from the lungs, thus helping to prevent and treat colds.

Low Immunity

Do cold and flu germs seem to make a beeline directly to you? When others fend off the sniffles easily, are you bedridden for days? Chances are your immune system could use some recharging.

> • *Herb at a Glance* •
> **Licorice.** Good for digestion, coughs, and respiratory congestion

The immune system is a complex network of organs, glands, and special cells that work in harmony to protect your body against infection and disease. It aggressively seeks and destroys viruses, bacteria, and other invaders. Most of the time, the immune system works perfectly well on its own. But if you're not well-nourished, well-rested, and prepared for daily stress, your immune system won't be strong enough to continuously fend off harmful intruders. As a consequence, you'll get sick often.

Bolster your immune system by eating right (five to seven servings of fruits and vegetables daily, as part of an eating plan that also emphasizes whole grains and low-fat protein sources), doing regular exercise (such as walking 30 minutes at least 5 days a week), getting sufficient rest (8 hours each night), and using stress management. Then add these herbal boosters.

Fortify with ginseng. Give your immune system a helping hand, especially during cold and flu season, with Siberian ginseng or panax ginseng (sometimes called Asian or Korean ginseng). Two or three times a day, take 40 to 60 drops of Siberian ginseng tincture mixed into a little water. Or try taking 20 to 40 drops of panax ginseng (often simply called ginseng on product labels) in water two or three times a day.

Studies show that Russian factory workers who used Siberian ginseng during cold and flu season took fewer sick days. Siberian ginseng contains substances that fuel the adrenal glands and help them to withstand emotional and physical stresses. It also contains compounds that fight viruses. Panax ginseng contains another group of compounds believed to stimulate immunity.

Enlist the immune system boosters. Help bolster your resistance to illness with the immune-strengthening powers of echinacea and other fortifying herbs. Combine ½ teaspoon each of tinctures of echinacea root, pau d'arco bark, Siberian ginseng root, licorice root, astragalus root, and bupleurum root. Take this mixture twice a day for a few weeks to fortify your immune system.

Arm germ-fighting cells with garlic. Fresh garlic cloves can be a faithful friend to an overworked immune system. Eat two cloves of fresh garlic every day. Garlic enhances your immune system by recharging your natural killer cells, white blood cells that seek and destroy disease-causing invaders. Mask the garlic odor by chewing on some parsley afterward.

Low Sexual Desire

Imagine desiring your partner so much that your heart flutters. Imagine feeling this passion—tonight. You can capture that "swept away" feeling, herbalists say, with the help of herbal oils and teas.

Inhale a sensual aroma. To set the mood for passion, scent your bedroom (or any room) with a few potent drops of sandalwood, rose, or amber essential oil. Just add a few drops of essential oil to a cup of warm water (the heat will release the aroma) or place five drops of essential oil and ½ cup of water in an atomizer, then shake and spray into the air. Sandalwood is a traditional aphrodisiac that makes you feel very centered in your body. Rose and amber have long had reputations for evoking sensuality.

Sip this love-enhancing tea. Boost blood circulation to the pelvic area with spicy, passion-producing tea. Simmer the following herbs in 2 cups of water for 20 minutes: 1 tablespoon of grated fresh ginger, 7 to 10 clove buds, 2 or 3 cinnamon sticks, 4 or 5 peppercorns, and 7 to 10 cardamom pods. Strain and add small amounts of milk and honey to taste. Top it with ¼ teaspoon of vanilla extract, a member of the orchid family known for being an aphrodisiac. Then enjoy this tea with your partner in a warm bath surrounded by beautiful candles. See where it leads.

Memory Problems and Poor Concentration

Ever find yourself rereading the same paragraph in a gripping mystery novel several times and still not recalling what it said? Do you tend to forget where you placed your car keys or find yourself in a supermarket aisle, unable to remember what you needed to buy? Ever blank out on a friend's name in the middle of an introduction?

Don't worry. Minor memory lapses and simple concentration slipups happen to everyone—they don't mean you're losing your memory. Forgetfulness and fuzzy thinking are often linked to stress, fatigue, and outright exhaustion.

Emotionally charged events, such as divorce, job loss, or the death of a loved one, can impair anyone's memory at any age. Stress causes the adrenal glands to release cortisol, a hormone that enables you to get through sudden emergencies. But over time, constant stress gradually kills or injures billions of brain cells, interfering with your ability to think and concentrate.

Once you've accounted for (and corrected) external factors that may be blunting your thinking, sharpen your memory and concentration further with these herbal helpers.

Give your brain a healthy workout with ginkgo. Improve bloodflow to the brain and enhance your brain's ability to use oxygen by taking 120 to 240 milligrams of ginkgo a day, divided into two doses. Dozens of studies in Germany and France have substantiated that ginkgo is an excellent

Jars of Memory Joggers

At the National College of Naturopathic Medicine in Portland, Oregon, students sometimes show up for class wearing wreaths of rosemary around their necks, especially when they're about to take a big test.

Is this some sort of herbal crib sheet? Or just a lucky charm, like a four-leaf clover or rabbit's foot? Not quite. According to Sharleen Andrews-Miller, a faculty member at the college, the scent of any of several common botanicals might be just the boost their brains need to keep their memories sharp. Those students know what they're doing!

Of course, most of us would prefer not to wear our herbs like a necklace, so something like a basil memory jar might be a better choice. Like rosemary, basil is thought to be a great brain booster. And kept in a jar, it will last longer, be easier to transport, and draw far less attention.

To make your own basil memory jar, stuff three or four cotton balls into a 1-ounce glass jar with a lid. Using a dropper, put 3 to 5 drops of basil essential oil into the jar, spreading the drops among the cotton balls. Screw the lid tightly onto the jar. When you need a memory or an alertness boost, open the jar and sniff the scent. Be sure to close the lid tightly so the essential oil doesn't dry out. Replace when the smell becomes faint.

herb for improving memory, especially for seniors. Make sure to select ginkgo tablets that are standardized to contain 24 percent ginkgo flavone glycosides and 6 percent terpene lactones—two of ginkgo's most important active ingredients.

Smell rosemary for remembrance. For minor concentration lapses and forgetfulness, sniff the scent of rosemary essential oil. Just apply 1 to 3 drops to a tissue, tuck it in your pocket, and inhale as needed. This herb's ability to improve memory and concentration dates back centuries. In fact, in Shakespeare's *Hamlet*, Ophelia declares, "There's rosemary, that's for remembrance."

Try a concentration-boosting formula. When you need to concentrate extra-hard for an important meeting or exam, this formula will improve your ability to focus. Combine 1 teaspoon each of tinctures of ginkgo and Siberian ginseng with ½ teaspoon each of tinctures of panax ginseng (also called Asian or Korean ginseng) and gotu kola. Take half a dropperful a few times a day and have an extra dose an hour before the big event.

Clinical studies show that these four herbs enhance mental abilities, including concentration, aptitude, alertness, and even intelligence.

Menopause

Today, as baby boomers move into midlife by the millions, menopause is recognized as a normal stage in life and not a disease. Many regard menopause as puberty in reverse, a time when you finally no longer need to worry about menstrual periods or birth control.

Strictly speaking, menopause means that you haven't had a menstrual period for a year, but well before that happens, you'll experience many changes. Since puberty, your body has amply produced the female hormones estrogen and progesterone. But by age 50, smaller and smaller amounts of these hormones are secreted, so eventually menstruation ceases.

As hormone production dwindles, you may experience

hot flashes, insomnia, irregular bleeding, mood swings, vaginal dryness, and other changes. Every woman experiences a unique combination of physical and emotional changes during this transition time.

Conventional medicine treats menopause as a deficiency disease of estrogen. Although doctors often prescribe hormone-replacement therapy (HRT), replacement hormones can't fully mimic your body's natural cycle. And some women stop taking HRT after experiencing the side effects, which can include menstrual-like bleeding, bloating, irritability, cramps, headaches, and depression.

Natural alternatives can help minimize menopausal symptoms. Consuming 30 to 50 milligrams each day of isoflavones, found in soy foods such as tofu, soy milk, and tempeh, seems to blunt bothersome hot flashes and vaginal dryness. Isoflavones are weak, plant-derived forms of estrogen. Engaging in regular aerobic activity helps combat weight gain, heart disease, and osteoporosis, conditions for which a woman's risk increases following menopause. Experts recommend that you exercise for at least 30 minutes two or three times a week (walking is ideal).

Besides dietary and lifestyle changes, certain herbs can protect your health as you go through menopause.

Try a combination blend. If you experience several change-of-life symptoms, look for multi-herb products formulated specifically for menopause. These usually contain some combination of the following strengthening and hormone-balancing herbs: chasteberry, black cohosh, dong quai, panax ginseng (also called Asian or Korean ginseng), and licorice root. These herbs balance and complement one another,

> • *Herb at a Glance* •
> **Mullein.** Good for bronchitis, coughs, and ear infections

which enhances their effectiveness and reduces side effects. For the most consistent results, look for blends that contain standardized extracts.

Stop mood swings with skullcap. Counter uncontrollable crying, angry outbursts, or other mood swings associated with menopause by taking skullcap twice a day. Use 4 to 8 drops of skullcap tincture every morning and evening when you feel fried, stressed-out, wired, or just wound up. Skullcap strengthens the nerves, eases sensitivity, and helps promote deep, sound sleep.

Cool hot flashes with black cohosh. Research shows that black cohosh, an herb that was used traditionally by Native Americans, is as effective as estrogen for the relief of hot flashes. To find the best dosage, herbalists suggest starting with 10 drops of black cohosh tincture twice a day and increasing the dose by 5 drops every other day until you're satisfied with the results. You may take it, as needed, for 2 weeks out of every month.

Menstrual Cramps and Bloating

Cramps are the result of a release of hormones called prostaglandins that cause uterine blood vessels to tighten, reducing bloodflow. This makes the uterine muscle flex in what you feel as a painful cramp. As for bloating, blame it on a drop in the female hormone progesterone in the 7 to 10 days before your menstrual cycle. Depletion of progesterone causes salt and water retention throughout your body.

Herbalists offer these botanical remedies that regulate hormones so that cramping and bloating become less severe.

Stop cramps quickly with cramp bark and valerian. If you're suffering from intense cramps and need relief right now, herbalists suggest blending 3 teaspoons of cramp bark tincture and 5 teaspoons of valerian tincture. Then take between 40 drops and 1 teaspoon of this blend in small amounts of warm water up to three times a day if necessary. Cramp bark relaxes muscles and soothes painful spasms. Valerian contains compounds that relieve muscle spasms and curb anxiety.

Ease pain with black haw. If menstrual cramps leave you doubled over in pain, herbal experts advocate taking black haw before pain peaks. This herb contains an aspirin-like compound that lessens the pain. Make a tea by adding 2 teaspoons of dried black haw to 1 cup of water. Boil for 10 minutes, cool, and strain. Drink up to 3 cups a day. It's best to start taking this tea a few days before you expect your period—don't wait until the pain becomes overwhelming.

Dodge discomfort with tea. Some women can lessen or even prevent menstrual cramps by drinking a hormone-balancing blend. To make the tea, combine one-quarter part dried chasteberry with one part each of dried wild yam, ginger, and yellow dock. Add two parts each of dried dandelion root, burdock, licorice, and sassafras. Brew the tea by adding 6 tablespoons of the blend to a quart of cold water in a pot. Simmer slowly for 20 minutes, then strain. Drink 3 to 4 cups daily for 3 weeks during each menstrual cycle, then stop while you menstruate. Long-term use of sassafras is not recommended; do not take more than the recommended dose.

These herbs help keep the liver healthy, an organ that is key to a woman's reproductive health. They promote bile flow so the liver can better process hormones. This blend also improves circulation, aids digestion, and fights uterine pain and cramping.

Halt bloating with dandelion. Dandelion leaves, a potent diuretic, effectively reduce uncomfortable bloating and swelling before and during menstruation. This herb also helps cleanse and rejuvenate the liver and promotes healthy digestion. Check with your naturopathic physician for availability and dosage.

Menstrual Flow, Heavy

Slight changes in your monthly menstrual flow are normal and may be brought on by lifestyle changes, such as starting a new job, beginning a new exercise routine, or moving into a new home. Age could also be a factor. Until around age 35, your uterus keeps growing, so there's more uterine lining to shed during menstruation. But as you approach menopause, in your forties and fifties, monthly periods can become unpredictable. Heavy bloodflow can drain your energy, lower your blood pressure, and intensify menstrual cramps.

Doctors urge you to pay attention to your monthly cycle so you know what's normal for you. Jot down when your period starts and ends. Record your bloodflow as heavy, medium, or light. It's especially important to see your doctor if heavy bleeding makes you feel light-headed, if you start passing blood clots, or if the heavy flow soaks through a pad or tampon every hour for 12 to 24 hours. Heavy bleeding that comes on suddenly may signal a miscarriage. Extra blood loss may also lead to anemia, an iron deficiency condition that makes you feel weak and weary.

After your physician rules out possible underlying medical causes for your heavy bleeding, herbalists recommend a two-prong strategy. Select some herbs to slow and regulate the flow and others to help correct hormone imbalances that can cause heavy bleeding.

Seek relief from yarrow and the gang. Stop an episode of excessive menstrual bleeding with the astringent herbs shepherd's purse, yarrow, geranium root, and lady's-mantle. Herbalists recommend a formula that combines two parts of shepherd's purse tincture with one part each of the tinctures of yarrow, geranium, and lady's-mantle. Take ½ to 1 teaspoon three or four times a day when menstrual flow is heavy.

Come to the aid of your liver. You can help correct hormone imbalances by feeding your liver, which processes certain hormones. Burdock, dandelion, fennel, and milk thistle are traditionally used for liver support. Milk thistle, the subject of more than 300 studies, contains silymarin, a substance that helps protect liver cells from toxic chemicals and at the same time stimulates the growth of new liver cells.

Create your own hormone-balancing, liver-friendly formula by using one or two of the following dried herbs: dandelion, milk thistle, burdock, or fennel. Brew a tea using 1 teaspoon of herb or herb mix per cup of boiling water, steep for 15 to 20 minutes, and strain. Have 2 to 3 cups a day. If a cup of tea isn't your cup of tea, you can take one 200-milligram milk thistle capsule two or three times a day. Or you can combine equal parts of the tinctures of your chosen liver herbs and have 1 teaspoon of the mix three times a day. Take liver-friendly herbs for several months.

Menstrual Period Irregularity

A woman's menstrual cycle doesn't always run on schedule. Illness, stress, travel, and aging can cause month-to-month fluctuations. For example, women in their twenties tend to have longer cycles, while women over 35 usually have shorter cycles because of hormonal changes.

At the start of a normal menstrual cycle, hormones prompt one or more eggs in the ovary to mature. By midcycle, one egg bursts from its follicle and sails down the Fallopian tube into the uterus. If it is fertilized during the

---

• *Herb at a Glance* •

Nettle. Good for allergy and hay fever symptoms

---

journey, a pregnancy begins. If not, menstruation starts. While some say this sequence of events normally occurs over 28 days, medical experts say the reality is that normal menstrual cycles for women can range in length from 21 to 38 days.

Be sure to discuss your menstrual cycle with your gynecologist during your yearly visit just to be certain everything is normal. If your cycle is truly irregular—dramatically shorter one month, longer the next—then these herbal remedies may help restore regularity.

Feed your reproductive system with a tonic tea. Take steps to regulate your cycle by first nourishing your reproductive system with a female tonic tea. This refreshing vitamin- and mineral-rich tea contains raspberry leaf, nettle, peppermint, and other herbs.

Make this tea by mixing two parts each of dried raspberry leaf, nettle, peppermint leaf, and lemongrass (for flavor) with one part each of dried strawberry leaf and lady's-mantle. Add a pinch of stevia to sweeten the mixture, if desired. Brew the tea by adding 6 tablespoons of the mix to a quart of cold water in a saucepan. Bring to a boil. Remove from the heat and steep for 20 minutes. Strain the herbs and drink 3 to 4 cups a day.

Get back on track with chasteberry. If hormonal imbalances turn the anticipated arrival date of your next monthly period into a guessing game, try restoring your schedule with chasteberry. This herb is commonly prescribed in Europe to regulate menstrual cycles.

Chasteberry, sometimes called vitex, seems to work through the pituitary gland, your body's master gland, to help reestablish hormonal balance.

Take a dropperful of chasteberry tincture two or three times a day in a small glass of warm water for 6 to 8 weeks.

Stop this daily routine during menstruation and resume when bleeding has stopped. Your menstrual cycle should become more regular within 2 to 4 months.

Find sweet harmony with licorice root. For a sweet-tasting tea with a well-rounded hormone-balancing effect, blend licorice root with chasteberry. Some herbalists say licorice root regulates and normalizes hormone production. To make a tea blend, use ½ teaspoon each of dried chasteberry and licorice root. Simmer lightly for 15 minutes in 1 cup of water. Strain; drink 3 cups of tea a day for two to four menstrual cycles.

Midafternoon Slump

In offices and homes across the country—and the world—a whole lot of yawning, stretching, and fighting off of sleep (or giving in to it) begins at about 2:00 P.M. Welcome to midafternoon, a natural siesta time for your body and mind.

Between 1:00 and 5:00 P.M., your brain and body function on minimum power. Mental focus fades. Blood sugar levels drop. Nerves fray. It's a natural, human rhythm: Within each 24-hour cycle, your body has two natural sleep periods—a long one at night and a short one at midafternoon. Small wonder, then, that some societies simply shut down for a few hours of midafternoon repose each day. But while a brief afternoon snooze will often revive you, who has time?

These herbs may help restore your mental focus, balance your blood sugar levels, and soothe frazzled nerves.

Inhale a high-energy scent. For a natural midafternoon pick-me-up, inhale the scent of rosemary, orange peel, or peppermint essential oil. Shake 1 or 2 drops of your chosen scent onto a tissue. Hold it close to your nose and inhale. You can also use a diffuser, a pump that blows the essential oil's scent into the air. Put the diffuser on your desk in your office or in your living room at home and turn it on when you feel in need of a pick-me-up.

Revive your energy with a mint-family tea. If you're sluggish by midafternoon, reach for a cup of mint tea, not coffee. Peppermint, spearmint, and lemon balm, all members of the mint family, are known for their ability to restore energy. Use 1 teaspoon of your chosen dried herb per cup of boiling water. Steep for 5 to 15 minutes, covered. Lemon balm is a perfect choice for times when you feel tired yet stressed, herbalists say. If you find yourself tired every afternoon, make a Thermos of your tea in advance and sip it slowly throughout the day.

Level blood sugar with dandelion. To balance blood sugar levels—and avoid sudden energy slumps—drink a cup of dandelion root tea. Boil 1 heaping teaspoon of dried dandelion root in 1½ cups of water for 15 to 20 minutes. Then strain and sip.

Migraines

If most ordinary headaches feel like a jeweler's hammer tapping on your temples, then a migraine feels like a sledgehammer pounding on your cranium.

Migraines, the most painful and debilitating of headaches, may stick around for several hours or even several days, causing nausea, vomiting, loss of appetite, and extreme sensitivity to light and sound—in addition to intense head pain. Like hurricanes, these intense headaches often give warnings of their approach. About 30 minutes before a migraine kicks in, your vision may blur or you may see bright spots. Your thinking may become jumbled. You may also feel numbness or tingling along one side of your body.

Unlike tension headaches, which are caused by muscle contractions, migraines are caused by the contraction of veins. Women often experience them during their periods because of changing levels of the hormone estrogen.

If your headache problem has never been diagnosed by your doctor, it's best to have yourself checked. Headaches are sometimes symptoms of other problems.

Herbal remedies can help prevent migraines or reduce their frequency, say herbalists. Here's how.

Fight back with feverfew. If you're prone to migraines, you can get relief with a daily dose of feverfew. Take ½ teaspoon of feverfew tincture or 500 milligrams in capsule form once a day. Research demonstrates that even small amounts of feverfew can prevent the pain of these awful headaches.

Eat ginger daily. Keep blood vessels in good shape with this common kitchen spice. Ginger inhibits a substance that prevents your blood vessels from dilating. There are many ways to fit ginger into your daily eating plan, herbalists say. You can grate fresh ginger into juice, munch on Japanese pickled ginger (available at health food stores), use fresh or powdered ginger while cooking, or snack on crystallized ginger candy.

Motion Sickness

Seasickness is just one form of motion sickness. Planes, trains, buses, and automobiles can bring on the same kind of queasiness. Motion sickness strikes when your brain receives conflicting messages about what's happening to your body. Suppose you're on a vacation flight to Orlando when the plane suddenly encounters severe turbulence. Your eyes signal to your brain that it *looks* as if you're sitting still. But your inner ear (which plays a role in balance) senses movement and tells your brain that you're moving forward—fast. The resulting confusion can bring on that I'd-rather-be-dead feeling of nausea, plus vomiting, cold sweats, and headaches.

If you're prone to this uncomfortable and inconvenient condition, you don't have to decline travel invitations in order to avoid nausea. With the right herbs, you can enjoy the motion without the sickness.

Take along ginger. This spicy root is the top choice of herbalists for soothing upset stomachs and preventing motion sickness. Herbalists suggest you take two 500-milligram capsules of ginger about 30 minutes before departure and then one or two more capsules if symptoms begin to occur, about every 4 hours. Studies show ginger works better than dimenhydrinate, the active ingredient in over-the-counter motion sickness medications such as Dramamine. Researchers think that ginger works by decreasing stomach movements caused by motion sickness or by shutting down impulses to the brain that deliver messages about equilibrium.

Select peppermint. If ginger is not available, the next best motion sickness fighter is peppermint. Although not as effective as ginger, peppermint can also soothe your nausea. About an hour before your trip, make a peppermint tea by pouring just-boiled water over a tablespoon of fresh peppermint in a cup. Cover it to keep the volatile oils from escaping and let it stand for 5 minutes. Strain and drink.

Be sure to take along premade peppermint tea in your travel mug for a nausea-free trip.

Muscle Cramps

Muscle cramps are sudden, sharp, painful contractions of the muscle fibers. In healthy people, cramping often results from overexertion and dehydration—running a marathon, for example, or spending 5 hours gardening in the summer heat and forgetting to take water breaks. Dehydration can lead to an electrolyte imbalance, meaning that levels of minerals that help cells function normally—sodium, calcium, and potassium—go out of kilter.

Inactivity, such as sitting too long in one position, can also bring on muscle cramps. Sometimes, they occur when you're just lying in bed, though no one's sure why.

To unkink and relax a tightened muscle, gently massage the area that's cramped, slowly stretch it, and then drink water or a sports drink to rehydrate. These herbal remedies will also help to soothe the ache.

Re-mineralize with nettle. Nettle is rich in minerals that can effectively alleviate cramping. Take one capsule or 30 drops of nettle tincture three times per day until the pain goes away. Mix the tincture with water, juice, or tea. A typical capsule dosage is between 300 and 450 milligrams.

Fight the ache with willow. For effective pain relief, take ½ teaspoon of willow bark tincture mixed with juice, tea, or water. Willow bark contains salicin, an aspirin-like compound that naturally fights a wide variety of pain—from muscle cramps to headaches to arthritis. You can increase your dose to as much as 5 teaspoons if you choose white willow tincture, which has a lower salicin concentration.

Get relief with ginkgo. To improve bloodflow in your limbs, and especially to knotted muscles, take one 80-milligram capsule of ginkgo (24 percent standardized extract) twice daily. Natural healers say ginkgo is an excellent choice for improving circulation.

> **• Herb at a Glance •**
> **Peppermint.** Good for preventing indigestion and treating bad breath, gas, and nausea

Muscle Strains and Sprains

An afternoon of digging up plants, playing tennis or golf, or even painting the house can leave you with a wrenched ankle or back or with stiff, painful muscles the next morning.

A strain occurs when you pull or tear a muscle or tendon. A sprain happens when you pull or overstretch a ligament. In either case, pain and swelling are sure to occur.

With muscle injuries, quick treatment can make a real difference in healing by drastically reducing swelling, bruising, and further muscular damage. For first-aid, wrap some ice in a towel and hold it on the affected area. How

---

Cayenne Ointment for Muscle Pain

If muscle pain has you down, try some cayenne ointment, also known as capsaicin cream. You should feel a warming or burning sensation when you apply the ointment to your skin. That feeling tells you that the capsaicin, the active ingredient in cayenne (also known as ground red pepper), is working. Capsaicin depletes substance P, a chemical made by your body that transmits pain messages from your nerves to your spinal cord, says Jenny McFeely, a member of Britain's National Institute of Medical Herbalists and a professional member of the American Herbalists Guild, who is from Scottsdale, Arizona. By disrupting those messages, you lessen pain.

Most creams contain between .025 and .075 percent capsaicin. If you don't want to feel the burning sensation on your hands, wear disposable gloves when applying the cream. Don't use cayenne cream on broken or injured skin, and avoid getting it into your eyes.

long you keep it there depends on the size of the injured muscle. Small muscles, such as those in the calves and elbows, require 10- to 15-minute treatments. Large muscles, such as those in the back and thighs, require 20-minute treatments. Use ice up to six times a day, until the swelling goes down, the bruising fades, and half the pain is gone.

After applying ice to the strain or sprain, incorporate these herbal healers.

Melt away pain with an herbal compress. Combine 1 to 2 teaspoons of tincture of arnica or St. John's wort and 2 tablespoons of cold water in a bowl. Soak a soft cloth in the mixture and apply the compress to the injured muscle to promote healing and to lessen the pain.

Rub on arnica oil. To combat bruising and swelling, apply arnica gel or oil to the affected muscle once a day for up to 3 days.

Stop swelling with bromelain. Herbal healers say this natural anti-inflammatory speeds healing of damaged tissue. Take 500 milligrams three times daily between meals until the pain subsides.

Pamper with herbal helpers. After a serious sprain, strain, or even broken bone has been treated by a doctor, enhance your long-term recovery with this poultice-and-oil treatment. First, place one handful of fresh comfrey or plantain leaves and ½ cup of water in a blender. Mix into a thick slush. Spread the poultice on a gauze pad and place it, slush side down, over the injured area. You can then cover the poultice with rolled cotton gauze to keep it in place. Leave the poultice on for up to 1 hour to reduce swelling. Both comfrey and plantain have skin-healing properties.

After the poultice, you can apply the following herbal healing oil: Combine 2 ounces of St. John's wort essential oil, ⅛ teaspoon of lavender essential oil, 8 drops of marjoram essential oil, and 2 drops of chamomile essential oil. Add this formula to about ¼ cup of your favorite unscented massage oil or vegetable oil. Apply the oil to your skin over your injury as needed to enhance healing.

Nail Problems

Fingernails can get brittle, weak, and dull when they're parched. Overexposure to household detergents, cold, heat, and wind causes nails to dry and break easily, leaving them with jagged edges, ragged cuticles, and cracked surrounding skin. Prolonged and repeated contact with water is also hazardous to your nails. Nails expand when they absorb water, then contract as the water evaporates. As water moves in and out of the nails, they weaken and crack. In addition, simply getting older can increase the chances that your nails will become thin and brittle.

In the 1950s, calcium supplements and gelatin drinks were touted for growing stronger nails. These remedies don't work. Here's what today's natural healers and beauty experts recommend for healthy nails that resist chips and tears.

Rub in herb-fortified castor oil. For ripped or dry nails, rub a drop of castor oil into the cuticle of each nail every day. Castor oil is thick and moisturizing, and it contains lots of vitamin E, so it's like food for your fingernails. An added bonus: It makes your nails shiny. Add a drop or two of skin-friendly carrot seed, lavender, or sandalwood essential oil to a 2-ounce bottle of castor oil for improved results.

Dunk your nails in lavender and sandalwood. If your nails crack easily, strengthen them with an herbal soak. Combine 2 tablespoons of jojoba oil with 4 drops each of lavender and sandalwood essential oils. Soak your nails in this mixture for 10 minutes. Then gently buff your nails to stimulate circulation and bring out a healthy shine.

Dip in horsetail. Nourish, condition, and protect dry, dull, brittle nails with a horsetail-comfrey soak. Horsetail is rich in silica, a substance that strengthens nails, according to experts on natural beauty. Comfrey has been used traditionally by herbal healers to soothe and mend damaged skin, and it will come to the aid of the cracked, dry skin around your nails. Combine ½ teaspoon of dried horsetail with 1 teaspoon of comfrey in a cup of boiling water. Steep for 15 to 20 minutes and let cool to a comfortable temperature. Then soak your nails in the mixture for 5 to 10 minutes. Repeat several times a week.

Nausea

An effective way to treat nausea is to give it the heave-ho—by throwing up. Vomiting is your body's way of getting rid of something it doesn't want sticking around any longer.

But sometimes, whether you've vomited or not, nausea lingers, and your stomach churns and cramps. You may even feel feverish. Although most stomach upsets depart on their own within 24 hours, here are some herbs to try for fast, stomach-soothing relief.

Grab some ginger. Touted as the top herb for just about all types of stomach upsets, ginger relieves nausea as well as dizziness. Ginger in capsule form is strongest, so it has the greatest medicinal effect. The recommended dose is one to two capsules three times per day for as long as you feel under the weather. (A typical dosage is 550 milligrams per capsule.) Or make a hot drink: Buy fresh gingerroot and cut off a slice about as long as your index finger. Simmer it in 2 cups of hot water for 15 minutes, then drink the liquid.

Improve digestion with dandelion. Ease nausea by aiding liver and digestive functions with this common

THE HERBAL KITCHEN

Say Goodbye to Tummy Aches

When that queasy, uneasy sensation of nausea unsettles your stomach, you want something that will bring relief quickly. Make a batch of this tonic and keep it on hand for moments of digestive distress, says Jenny McFeely, a member of Britain's National Institute of Medical Herbalists and a professional member of the American Herbalists Guild, who is from Scottsdale, Arizona. This mixture contains herbs that aid digestion and relax and calm the stomach.

¼ ounce black horehound tincture or extract
¼ ounce meadowsweet tincture or extract
¼ ounce anise tincture or extract
¼ ounce German chamomile tincture or extract
25 drops ginger tincture or extract

In a 1-ounce or larger bottle with a dropper lid, mix the black horehound, meadowsweet, anise, and chamomile. Then add the ginger. Shake well. Take 5 to 8 drops of the tonic as needed.

backyard herb. Take one capsule, which typically contains about 520 milligrams, or 30 drops of dandelion root tincture with meals. If taking the tincture, squeeze it into ¼ cup of water and sip it slowly until it's gone. Do this three times a day.

Boot out nausea with meadowsweet. A cup of meadowsweet tea can make that tummy feel better. Meadowsweet soothes inflammation, calming your system and reducing nausea. Use 1 tablespoon of the dried herb per cup of just-boiled water. Steep for 5 to 10 minutes before straining out the herb. Then take tiny sips.

Nicotine Withdrawal

Anyone who has ever tried to stop smoking, successfully or not, has paid a visit to hell.

Even though you've tossed the cigarettes, stashed the ashtrays, and announced to all your friends and family that cigarettes will never again touch your lips, you still want nicotine. In fact, you don't just want it. You *crave* it.

The truth is, cigarettes are just as addictive as cocaine or even heroin, and they're equally hard to ditch. More than one-third of people who try to stop smoking report significant withdrawal symptoms: irritability, anxiety, hunger, fatigue, dry mouth, headaches, insomnia, constipation, and, of course, the need for a cigarette.

But remember, nicotine withdrawal is only temporary. You *can* get through it. By contrast, a lifetime of smoking can lead to permanent problems: cancer, heart attacks, strokes, osteoporosis, fertility problems, and early menopause.

Doctors say that exercise relieves irritability and anxiety and helps you avoid adding extra pounds when you quit smoking. Snacking on low-calorie foods such as carrot sticks, apples, and even sugarless gum helps, too. Herbs can also contribute to an easier, more peaceful transition to a smoke-free life. Consider these botanical options.

Clear your throat and calm your mind with a three-herb tea. Especially during your first few days without cigarettes, you may feel jittery and need to get rid of excess phlegm in your lungs. This anti-smoking herbal tea helps both problems. Blend equal amounts of dried chamomile, dried skullcap, and dried catnip, and then add 2 teaspoons of this mix per cup of just-boiled water. Steep up to 30 minutes, strain, and drink ¼ cup four times per day. Chamomile is a gentle relaxant, as is skullcap, which has also been used to treat drug and alcohol addiction. Catnip, another relaxant, has been used traditionally for respiratory ailments.

Overcome nicotine withdrawal with oats and more.
Calm withdrawal symptoms with this botanical formula suggested by natural healers. Combine ½ teaspoon each of the tinctures of valerian and skullcap, 1 teaspoon of tincture of fresh oats, and ½ teaspoon each of the tinctures of St. John's wort and passionflower. Take 2 to 5 dropperfuls of the mixture daily. Practitioners of Ayurvedic medicine have been recommending oats for at least 1,000 years to treat opium addiction. Recent studies have shown that a tincture made from oats can also help people stop smoking. The other herbs in this formula are calming and uplifting.

Reach for a cigarette substitute. If you miss holding a cigarette between your fingers or your lips, switch from cigarettes to a sweet stick of licorice root. Herbalists aren't sure how it works, but licorice root somehow satisfies oral cravings that people who are addicted to cigarettes seem to have. Don't substitute licorice candy, however, since it rarely contains real licorice.

Night Sweats

Night sweats are nocturnal hot flashes. Unpredictable and uncomfortable, these symptoms of menopause can wake you from a sound sleep and leave you drenched in perspiration.

Medical experts aren't sure what causes night sweats, but they seem to be linked to the hormonal changes that occur before and during menopause. It may be that your body's heat regulation system gets thrown off when hormones are in flux. Or it may be that hormonal changes irritate blood vessels and nerves, causing the blood vessels to overdilate, making you feel hot. In any case, night sweats interrupt sleep and can leave you irritable and depressed during the day.

For comfort, sleeping in all-cotton pajamas on all-cotton sheets is recommended. Synthetics or blends that trap body heat can trigger a night sweat. Also, keep a carafe of ice water on your nightstand to sip. During an episode, taking slow, deep breaths can help. And finally, you can turn to herbs.

Have a cool herbal soak. Reduce the frequency and severity of night sweats by cooling off in an herbal bath before going to bed. Put the following essential oils into ½ cup of carrier oil, such as grapeseed, almond, or apricot: 4 drops of chamomile, 6 drops of lemon, and 10 drops of evening primrose. Then dump the mixture into a tub of comfortably warm—not hot—water. Soak in the bath long enough for the water to cool, usually about 20 minutes. Chamomile is said to relax the body, lemon cools and calms, and evening primrose aids hormonal balance.

Rely on motherwort. To subdue night sweats, herbalists suggest motherwort. Dilute 5 to 15 drops of tincture of motherwort, made from fresh, flowering tops, in a little water or tea. Take as needed.

Act fast with sage. For quick results, stave off night sweats with garden sage. Make this tea in advance and keep it by your bedside: Add 4 heaping tablespoons of dried sage to 1 cup of hot water. Cover tightly and steep for 4 hours or more, then strain it. Sage is useful for menopause because of its estrogenic action and because it dries up perspiration.

Oily Hair

Contrary to popular belief, "problem" oily hair doesn't exist. The problem is not your hair. It's your scalp.

Oil on your scalp, just like the oil on your skin, comes from sebaceous glands. Attached to hair follicles, these sacs secrete sebum, a mixture of fatty acids, which prevents the scalp from drying out. Excess sebum weighs in-

Make Your Own Herbal Shampoo

Why buy expensive herbal shampoo when you can make your own? This shampoo gently cleans yet doesn't strip away your hair's natural oils, and it doubles as an herbal body wash, says Mindy Green, a founding and professional member of the American Herbalists Guild and director of educational services for the Herb Research Foundation in Boulder, Colorado.

To pick your herbs and essential oils, Green offers the following suggestions.

- For dry hair: Use the herb orange peel, calendula, or comfrey. Use the essential oil sandalwood or rosewood.
- For oily hair: Use the herb sage, lemongrass, burdock, or lemon peel. Use the essential oil clary sage, lemongrass, patchouli, cypress, or cedarwood.

dividual hairs down. As a consequence, your hair looks flat, dull, and lifeless.

Here are some herbal ways to keep excessive sebum production from masking your hair's natural beauty.

Make your own shampoo. If you can't locate a commercial shampoo that keeps your hair from looking oily, concoct your own. Just add 4 drops each of rosemary and lavender essential oils to 2 ounces of any unscented shampoo. Shake the mixture well, then wash your hair as usual. Start off with a quarter-size dollop, adjusting the amount to the length of your hair. Both rosemary and lavender essential oils control oiliness and add shine to your hair. Essential oils can irritate, so don't get this shampoo in your eyes. And if you notice any skin irritation, stop using it.

- For all types: Use the herb lavender, chamomile, rosemary, or rose. Use the essential oil lavender, Roman chamomile, rosemary, or carrot seed.
- For dandruff: Use the herb burdock, sage, or willow bark. Use the essential oil sage, geranium, juniper, cedarwood, or tea tree.

To make the shampoo, purchase an empty 4-ounce shampoo bottle at a beauty supply store. (Limiting each batch to 4 ounces ensures freshness.) Using a funnel, pour in 2 ounces of an unscented shampoo base, which can be bought at a beauty supply or health food store. Make 2 ounces of a strong infusion or decoction of your chosen herb. Let cool, strain, and mix with the shampoo base. Add 30 drops (¼ teaspoon) of your selected essential oils. Shake well before each use.

Improve your commercial shampoo with essential oils. If you love your store-bought shampoo, simply enhance it with this herbal formula: Dilute an 8-ounce bottle of shampoo by half with water and add about 20 drops of the essential oil of lavender, lemongrass, or patchouli. Regular shampooing with this mild, herb-rich formula will keep your oil glands under control.

Finish with an herbal rinse. To complete your hair-washing regimen, herbalists suggest this oil-fighting herbal rinse. Pour 1 pint of boiling water over 1 teaspoon each of the dried herbs burdock root, calendula flowers, chamomile flowers, lavender flowers, lemongrass, and sage leaves. Steep for about 30 minutes. Strain, and add 1 tablespoon of vinegar. Pour this herbal mix over your scalp and hair as a final rinse after shampooing. For best results, don't rinse it out. The herbs discourage excess oil production, while the vinegar helps prevent dandruff.

Oily Skin

Ah, the oily skin dilemma: Oil makes noses shine and chins glisten, but it also makes skin soft, supple, and less likely to wrinkle.

Blame excess oil on overeager sebaceous glands, tiny derricks that can sometimes pump out a little more lubrication than most of us want or need. You may try to dispel excess oil with strong soaps and astringents. But natural beauty experts say they may be too harsh on your skin, and stripping too much oil away may simply signal your sebaceous glands to produce more.

Strike a healthy balance with these herbal remedies.

Gently conquer overactive oil glands with strawberry and lavender. Make oily skin feel clean and oil-free with a strawberry-lavender clay mask, herbal beauty experts suggest. Make the mask by combining 1 tablespoon of facial clay (available at health food stores), 1 tablespoon of witch hazel, one mashed strawberry, and one drop of lavender essential oil. Apply to your face, avoiding the area around your eyes. Leave it on for 10 to 15 minutes, then rinse with warm water. Strawberry helps normalize overactive oil glands, while lavender calms the central nervous system.

Steam open pores. To unclog pores and eliminate excess oil, steam your face with water and herbs at least once a week. Simmer 3 cups of water in a pan. Then add 1 heaping teaspoon each of chamomile, lemongrass, lavender, and rosemary. Remove from the heat and steep for 5 minutes. Set the pan in a place where you can comfortably sit next to it. Create a mini-sauna by covering the back of your head with a towel and tucking the ends around the pan. Hold your head about 12 inches away from the water. Make sure that the steam is not so hot that it feels uncomfortable. Be sure to keep your eyes closed so the oils don't sting. Remain in the steam for a few minutes, then come out to cool your face. Do this a few times.

The herbs will encourage your oil glands to function more normally.

Osteoporosis

Osteoporosis leaves bones weak, brittle, and porous. It may show no outward symptoms for years—which explains why more than 25 million Americans, among them many postmenopausal women, don't even know they have osteoporosis until they sustain a fracture. Women are at particular risk after menopause because production of the female hormone estrogen sharply declines. Estrogen helps bones absorb and retain calcium. But men are also prey to osteoporosis.

Bone loss actually starts much earlier in life. After age 35, you'll lose a little every year. In 20 years, you'll be down by 10 to 20 percent. You can slow that loss down, or even add some bone, with regular exercise, calcium supplements, and herbs. Medical experts recommend at least 30 minutes of weight-bearing exercise (such as jogging or weight lifting) every day as well as walking at least 30 minutes three times a week. In addition, supplement your diet with at least 1,200 milligrams of calcium and 300 to 500 milligrams of magnesium daily. Then complete your anti-osteoporosis strategy with these helpful herbs.

Maximize calcium intake with gentian. Ensure that calcium is properly absorbed from food and vitamin supplements by taking one capsule of gentian root before each meal (a typical capsule is 550 milligrams). This herb prompts stomach acids to effectively break down calcium so that it can be absorbed more completely.

Reduce your risk with horsetail. Horsetail is among the richest plant sources of silicon, a mineral that helps prevent osteoporosis and can be used to treat bone fractures, according to French studies. Natural healers suggest taking up to nine 350-milligram capsules of horsetail per day, but consult with a holistic practitioner to find the proper dose for you.

You can also take horsetail in tea form by adding about 1 tablespoon of dried horsetail and 1 teaspoon of sugar to each cup of water you use. Bring to a boil in a pan, then simmer for about 3 hours. Strain the leaves. Allow the tea to cool before drinking. (The sugar pulls more silicon from the herb.)

Appreciate avocados. For an added bone fortifier, sprinkle black pepper generously on avocados. Black pepper contains four anti-osteoporosis compounds. Avocado is loaded with bone-healthy vitamin D and heart-healthy vitamin E. Try mashing an avocado into calcium-rich nonfat cottage cheese or yogurt and sprinkling black pepper on top.

Overweight

If there really were a magic weight-loss pill, we'd all stock our shelves with it—and own stock in the company that makes it. There isn't, and we don't. Natural healers and conventional practitioners alike still give the same advice: The most effective natural solution for unwanted pounds is a combination of healthy diet and regular exercise.

Eat more foods high in fiber, such as fruits, vegetables, beans, potatoes, and whole grains. Fiber gives you the feeling of being full and stabilizes blood sugar levels. In addition, make time for at least 30 minutes of aerobic exercise 5 to 7 days a week. Walking counts, as does any other activity that gets your heart pumping faster and your lungs

A No-Cal Substitute for Your Sweet Tooth

Does this sound anything like you? Barbara has been trying to lose the same 30 pounds for years. She blames her sweet tooth. She seems to crave something sugary several times a day. Recently, she discovered stevia, a super-sweet herb that comes in dried or liquid form. She adds it to everything—iced tea, hot tea, cereal, baked goods. Has Barbara found the answer to her craving for sugar?

Perhaps, says Emily Kane, N.D., a naturopathic physician in Juneau, Alaska. Of course, Barbara would be better off with foods that don't need sweetening. But she's not likely to give up sweets. That's where stevia comes in. Stevia, an herb from Paraguay, is as sweet as sugar but has no calories. (One teaspoon of sugar has 16 calories. Candy and cookies typically have a huge number of calories—and little nutritional value.)

Using stevia instead of sugar in her sweet treats still doesn't give Barbara much nutritional value, but she's cutting out quite a few calories. And stevia doesn't promote tooth decay, so she's doing her smile a favor as well. Barbara has made a good start, and she's benefiting from her switch to stevia in more ways than she probably realizes.

By modifying her diet and substituting stevia for sugar, she will probably lose a good bit of those extra 30 pounds. And she'll enjoy herself while she's doing it.

working harder, including running, bicycling, swimming, or taking an aerobics class. Remember to check with your doctor before starting any exercise program.

That said, don't discount herbs. Chosen and used with care, they can give a sensible weight-loss program an added advantage. Sometimes, they may even make all the difference between success and failure.

Rev up your metabolism with green tea. For a safe weight-loss herb, herbalists suggest drinking a cup of green tea with a meal two or three times per day. Or take two 170-milligram capsules three times per day. Green tea contains caffeine and theobromine, both of which are stimulants. "So why don't I just drink a cup of coffee?" you might ask. Green tea has nutritional advantages that coffee doesn't, including vitamin C and flavonoids, potent antioxidants that reduce the risk of illnesses such as heart disease and colon cancer.

If you're trying to cut back on caffeine, though, don't have more than 2 cups of green tea per day.

Sprinkle cayenne on your food. If you're trying to lose weight, call on cayenne pepper (also known as ground red pepper), which raises your metabolic rate and stimulates thirst. If you fill up on water instead of food, you'll take in fewer calories and gain less weight. Add a dash of cayenne pepper to your food several times per day. In research conducted at Oxford Polytechnic Institute in England, dieters who added 1 teaspoon of cayenne pepper and 1 teaspoon of mustard to every meal raised their metabolic rates by as much as 25 percent.

Shed pounds with a five-star herb formula. Here's a gentle blend that can help you to lose pounds and improve your metabolism. Blend the following tinctures in a bottle: 1 ounce of nettle, 1 ounce of dandelion leaf, 1 ounce of bladderwrack, 2 ounces of guggul, and 2 ounces of schisandra berry. All are available at health food stores. Take ½ to 1 teaspoon three times per day. Hold your nose before you drink, however, because this isn't the most pleasant-tasting of concoctions.

Nettle is loaded with minerals that help maintain overall health. Dandelion aids the liver in secreting bile, which helps break down fats. Bladderwrack is a folk remedy for being overweight. Guggul helps normalize thyroid function, which is sometimes disturbed in overweight people. Schizandrin, the active ingredient in schisandra berry, stimulates metabolism.

Perimenopause

For women in their midforties to late fifties, perimenopause can be a frustrating and confusing gray zone. You're on the brink of menopause—as if you're standing at the very edge of a diving board, about to leap in—yet you're still not completely finished with menstruation.

Usually, the first signs of perimenopause are irregular or shorter menstrual cycles. The female hormone estrogen (and sometimes progesterone) starts to cycle at lower levels. The uterus reacts by shedding its lining early or off-schedule. In addition, some women experience symptoms that are similar to those of menopause: hot flashes, night sweats, insomnia, vaginal dryness, heart palpitations, depression, anxiety, and forgetfulness.

As a result, many botanical solutions recommended for perimenopause by herbalists and naturopaths are the same as those suggested for menopause. Let these herbs assist you during this transitional time in life.

Rely on black cohosh. For relief from most of the discomforts this time of life may bring you, especially hot flashes, anxiety, and vaginal dryness, try black cohosh. The recommended dosage is a 40-milligram capsule (containing a standardized extract of 2.5 to 2.6 percent triterpene glycosides) two to four times daily. Clinical studies suggest that it can relieve many perimenopausal symptoms.

Balance hormones with chasteberry. To even out hormonal imbalances at perimenopause, natural healers recommend chasteberry (also known as vitex). If you have irregular periods, take a dropperful of chasteberry tincture in a small glass of water or juice two or three times per day for 6 to 8 weeks. This shrub has been studied extensively and has been proven to relieve hot flashes, dizziness, and menstrual irregularities. Chasteberry influences the pituitary gland to slow down secretion of the hormone prolactin, which helps to normalize irregular menstrual cycles.

Enjoy soy. To fight hot flashes, balance estrogen, and protect against uterine and breast cancer, take 50 milligrams of soy-extract isoflavones two or three times per day. In nations where women eat soy products regularly, perimenopausal symptoms are less severe.

PMS

Some women jokingly refer to premenstrual syndrome (PMS) as pity-me syndrome. But PMS is no joke, and it is relief—not pity—that women with it seek.

The monthly discomfort of PMS strikes 8 out of every 10 women. Some weep without reason. Others blow their stacks or experience unstoppable food cravings. Still others complain of bloating, headaches, and acne breakouts. All told, PMS has more than 150 possible symptoms.

The cause behind PMS is still unknown. Some scientific studies indicate that some women with PMS possess below-normal levels of serotonin, a mood-regulating brain chemical. Another theory links PMS to fluctuating levels of estrogen and progesterone, both female hormones.

With its many symptoms, PMS isn't a simple condition to relieve. Top herbalists work with women to create customized PMS formulas to match their specific needs. Generally, they choose herbs that help balance hormones, stop mood swings, and improve liver function, which helps your body to eliminate excess hormones more effectively. Over a period of months, these herbal treatments can help your body function in a healthier way and free you from many of the challenges PMS can offer. Here are some herbs to try.

Chase away PMS with chasteberry. Chasteberry (also known as vitex) can give you a great head start on coping with PMS. To make a tea, use 1 teaspoon of the dried herb per cup of boiling water. Steep for 20 minutes, strain, then drink up to 3 cups per day. Studies show that chasteberry extract relieves end-of-cycle symptoms in women more effectively than vitamin B_6, a time-honored PMS remedy. Herbal experts say chasteberry seems to work by elevating levels of progesterone, the female hormone that rules the second half of the menstrual cycle.

Deflate bloating with yarrow. When PMS causes your abdomen to swell, reverse bloating with yarrow, herbal healers suggest. Combine one-half part dried yarrow and one part dried chasteberry to make a tea. Then use 1 teaspoon of this mix per cup of boiling water. Steep for 20 minutes, strain, and sip up to 3 cups daily. A mild diuretic, yarrow also stimulates the liver, which helps balance hormones.

Pacify PMS moods with aromatherapy. To fend off anger or anxiety, rely on aromatherapy to put you in a better mood. For anger, dab 2 drops of rose and 3 drops of sandalwood essential oils on a handkerchief and smell it. For anxiety, try sniffing the scent of sandalwood, ylang-ylang, or orange blossom essential oil.

Poison Ivy, Poison Oak, and Poison Sumac

"Leaves of three, let it be." Maybe your grandpa taught you this warning the first time you hiked in the woods with him. It's good advice if you don't want to leave the

Poison Plants and Their Antidotes

If poison ivy, oak, or sumac caresses your exposed skin while you're hiking, search the roadsides and woodland edges for jewelweed.

Scientists have discovered that jewelweed contains a chemical called lawsone. This substance blocks the action of urushiol, the plant resin that causes the allergic reaction. If applied quickly after contact with a poison plant, lawsone locks out urushiol and prevents rashes from developing.

Grab a bunch of jewelweed (leaves and stems), crush it into a ball in your hands, and rub your skin with its juice, says Ellen Evert Hopman, a professional member of the American Herbalists Guild from Amherst, Massachusetts, and author of *Tree Medicine, Tree Magic* and *A Druid's Herbal for the Sacred Earth*. Jewelweed has orange flowers and blue-green, spoon-shaped leaves. If you can find them, use the reddish protuberances, which are actually rootlets, on the lower stem of jewelweed. These may contain the highest concentrations of lawsone. Squeeze the liquid out of the rootlets onto a tissue or directly onto the rash. It may take a few plants to get enough of the liquid.

You're most likely to find jewelweed in moist, shaded areas. This tall plant often grows alongside poison ivy,

woods itchy. That old-time saying reminds you to avoid contact with poison ivy. But you should also steer clear of poison oak and poison sumac.

Poison ivy thrives in ankle-deep ground cover, especially on the East Coast. Poison oak is more common to the West Coast. Poison sumac is a shrub or small tree with white berries common in swampy areas of the East Coast.

since both plants are prolific weeds. Be sure to carefully choose leaves that are farthest from any nearby poison ivy plants to eliminate any exposure to the ivy's irritating oils. Look for the orange-flowered variety, not the yellow. The orange flowers bloom from June to September.

Here's how to recognize the poison plants.

Poison ivy grows as a shrub or vine. The plant has three shiny leaves—the middle leaf is bigger—connected to one stem. The leaves are reddish in the spring, green in the summertime, and various shades of red, orange, yellow, or bronze in the fall. The plant's tiny yellow-green flowers grow in clusters.

Poison oak can reach a height of 6½ feet, and its stems are slender and woody. Look for clusters of three rounded leaves that resemble oak leaves. Small white flowers with five petals grow on it in clusters.

Poison sumac is a tall shrub or small tree with 6 to 12 leaflets arranged in pairs, with a single leaflet at the end of each branch. The clustered flowers start out small and yellow-green but evolve into white-green fruits that hang on loose clusters 4 to 8 inches long. Nonpoisonous sumac grows red fruits on cone-shaped heads.

A few lucky people aren't allergic to urushiol, the thick, oily substance in the resin of these plants that provokes that annoying, itchy rash. Most of us, however, aren't so fortunate. Even indirect contact, such as handling clothing or shoes that have brushed against a poison plant or petting a dog or cat that just rolled in a poison ivy patch, can raise those itchy blisters on your skin.

> • *Herb at a Glance* •
> **Rosemary.** Good for
> preventing migraines
> and treating congestion
> and fever

This allergic reaction can also make you feel nauseated, tired, fuzzy-headed, and feverish. In severe cases, it can lead to unrelenting itching and infection, and sometimes the rash even spreads to the face or eyes. If you develop such a severe rash, see your doctor; you may need a corti-sone shot.

Milder cases respond well to herbal remedies. Before reaching for herbal relief, however, first carefully remove urushiol from your skin, medical experts advise. As soon as possible, wash thoroughly with soap or a strong deter-gent. (Fels Naptha soap works very well.) Remove all clothing and wash it. Then try these itch-stopping, rash-relieving herbal remedies.

Be prepared with grindelia. Before setting out on a hiking trip through the woods, plan ahead by packing a tincture of grindelia (also called gumweed) in your back-pack. Immediately after brushing up against a poisonous plant, wipe your exposed skin with grindelia tincture.

Nix the itch with an herbal paste. If you're already itching and sporting an oozing rash, soothe your skin with an herbal paste. Combine 2 tablespoons of grindelia or jew-elweed tincture and 2 tablespoons of comfrey tincture with 2 tablespoons of distilled water. Stir the liquid ingredients into ¼ cup of colloidal oatmeal (available in drugstores) or 1 to 2 tablespoons of bentonite clay until you form a paste. If colloidal oatmeal is not available, grind rolled oats in a coffee mill or blender. Apply to the affected skin. These herbs calm the itch and discourage oozing. Allow the paste to dry on your skin, and leave it on until you bathe.

Halt swelling with echinacea. Herbalists say you can soothe the inflammation of a poison-plant rash with an echinacea wash. Just mix one part echinacea tincture in three parts water. Use the wash on the affected skin several times per day. German research shows that echinacea helps reduce inflammation when applied externally.

Psoriasis

Television advertisements used to call it the heartbreak of psoriasis—and, indeed, the red rashes and silvery scales brought on by this skin condition are both unsightly and uncomfortable. Natural healers say the best way to soothe psoriasis is with a combination of remedies that work on the outside surface of the skin as well as others that work from inside of you.

In psoriasis, skin cells grow at an abnormal rate, often 1,000 times faster than normal. These cells pile up in clumps that look like silvery scales. Although unsightly red patches and scales can appear anywhere on your skin, they usually show up on your scalp, on the backs of your ears, on your elbows, or behind your knees.

Pinpointing the reason for this rapid cell division can be difficult, but medical experts say people with psoriasis usually have high levels of polyamine, a toxic amino acid that forms as a result of poor digestion. Stress also plays a role. More than one-third of people with psoriasis say their initial outbreak occurred within a month of a very stressful event. Outbreaks can also be provoked by injuries, infections, or a change of season. This skin condition may be inherited but is not contagious.

The first steps in psoriasis relief? Stop using soap. It will irritate sensitive skin. And try to get out in the sun for about an hour per day. Exposure to ultraviolet light slows down the abnormal growth of skin cells.

Natural healers also recommend specific herbs that soothe skin and improve liver function. They believe that when the liver can't process the toxins, hormones, fats, and other substances in the bloodstream completely, some toxins are sent to the skin to be eliminated. If these toxins irritate the skin, it worsens a psoriasis outbreak. Here are some ways to soothe psoriasis, on the surface and from deep within.

Cleanse with healing herbs. Instead of using soap, try this herbal cleanser especially designed for dry skin and psoriasis. Blend 2 ounces of aloe vera gel, 1 teaspoon of vegetable oil, 1 teaspoon of glycerin, ½ teaspoon of grapefruit seed extract, 8 drops of sandalwood essential oil, and 4 drops of rosemary essential oil. Shake well before each use. Apply with cotton balls to the affected skin areas, then rinse off. This cleanser fights inflammation and heals the irritation that develops as outer layers of dry skin flake off.

Rally 'round your liver with milk thistle or yellow dock. A tincture of yellow dock or milk thistle will boost liver function, natural healers note. Take 30 to 60 drops of either, in water, juice, or herbal tea, two or three times per day for up to 9 months. These traditional skin healers help the liver filter out toxins that irritate sensitive skin.

Puffy Eyes

Blame baggy under-eye pouches on too little sleep—or too many tears. Allergies, salty foods, and hormonal changes can also prompt your body to collect and retain fluid under your eyes.

Whatever the cause, walking around with puffy eyes is no picnic. Wraparound sunglasses help—when you're out in the sun. So do cover-up concealer creams—as long as they're not so light that they actually attract attention to your eyes. But instead of hiding those under-eye pouches, try these gentle herbal solutions to deflate them.

Ease away puffiness with fennel. If you're prone to puffy eyes, have this cool-comfort remedy ready to use. Pour a cup of boiling water over 2 teaspoons of fennel seeds and cover. Let steep, then put the whole pot in the refrigerator overnight. In the morning, strain the cooled tea, which should smell like licorice.

Cut paper towels into patches slightly larger than your eyes and soak them in the cool fennel tea. Lie down with your head elevated on a pillow. Cover your closed eyes with the patches. Rewet the patches whenever they warm up. Within 15 minutes, your eyes should look and feel better. This mixture lasts for 4 days when stored in the refrigerator.

Go with chamomile for quick relief. Rely on chamomile tea bags to unpuff those eyes, natural beauty experts say. Just close your eyes and lay wet, chilled chamomile tea bags over them for 10 to 20 minutes. Chamomile gently constricts blood vessels, which may help minimize puffiness. Don't use this remedy if you're allergic to pollen. You may react to the pollen-rich flower heads found in chamomile.

Restore bright eyes with dandelion. Gently flush excess fluid—which can cause under-eye puffiness—out of your body by drinking a cup or two of dandelion tea per day. To make the tea, use 1 teaspoon of dried dandelion leaf and 1 teaspoon of dried dandelion root per cup of boiling water. Steep in a teapot or covered pan for 10 minutes. Then strain and sip. Dandelion acts as a cleansing diuretic that reduces water retention. If you have gallbladder disease, don't use dandelion preparations without your doctor's approval.

Sinusitis

Sometimes, your body's air-filtration system goes on the fritz. Viruses, pollen, or polluted air can irritate and inflame the delicate mucous membranes lining your nasal passages, cutting off drainage from your sinus cavities.

The result is pressure and pain across your forehead and around your eyes and nose. You develop a stuffed-up, can't-breathe feeling. Sometimes, you get headaches. Your eyes may become red, itchy, and scratchy. If infection sets in, you may also develop a fever and experience nasal discharge.

Some people come down with sinusitis only occasionally. For others, it's a painful chronic condition. Along with decongestants, antibiotics are usually prescribed if an infection has flared up. If you have a fever, a puslike nasal discharge, or persistent pain, see your doctor. If your symptoms are less severe, consider the following botanical remedies, recommended by top herbalists.

Unclog with goldenseal. Soothe inflamed mucous membranes fast with goldenseal. Try 10 to 25 drops of goldenseal tincture mixed in water as often as five times per day. Goldenseal contains two active compounds that fight infection. Use this herb only until your sinus inflammation has cleared. It is not meant for long-term use.

Inhale congestion-clearing eucalyptus. Create a sinus-soothing steam with eucalyptus essential oil, herbalists suggest. Heat up some water on the stove until it boils, then pour it into a bowl. Add a couple of drops of eucalyptus essential oil. Drape a towel over your head and, keeping your face about 12 inches away from the water, breathe in the steam from the bowl for about 5 minutes. The humidity of the steam and the action of the essential oil work to loosen mucus and help you to breathe freely.

Tame sinus headaches with eyebright. To ease the pain of a sinus headache, herbalists recommend taking 5 milligrams of eyebright tincture, mixed in water, every 4 to 6 hours until the pain and infection disappear. This grasslike herb combines anti-inflammatory powers with an astringent action. Besides subduing sinus headaches, eyebright also helps to dry up congestion and runny noses.

Sore Throat

Marathon chats. Cigarette smoke. Cheering at a football game. A cold. A cough. An allergy. Any—and all—of these can leave your throat raw, scratchy, and inflamed.

Sore throats happen when the mucous membrane lining your airways dries out. The result? It hurts to swallow.

If you develop a sore throat with a fever but no other cold or allergy symptoms, you may have a strep infection, which requires medical attention. Should your doctor determine that you have strep throat, he will probably prescribe antibiotics.

But for routine sore throats, here's what nature has to offer.

Gargle away infection with soothing herbs. If your throat is infected and full of mucus, gargle with a tea made from dried sage, thyme, goldenseal, echinacea, or myrrh. Take a teaspoonful of your chosen herb, add 8 ounces of boiling water, let it steep in a covered container for 10 minutes, and strain. Allow it to cool to a comfortable temperature, then gargle with it as often as necessary. These herbs fight infection and reduce inflammation.

Suck on slippery elm. For dry, scratchy, sore throats, slippery elm lozenges can supply a steady stream of relief. Slippery elm is rich in soothing mucilage, which means it creates a little healthy mucus to help you expel whatever irritants are making you cough, and it protects irritated mucous membranes. It also acts as a mild cough suppressant.

THE HERBAL KITCHEN

Soothing Sore Throat Tea

Calm an irritated throat with this soothing tea, created by Angela Stengler, N.D., a naturopathic physician and herbal author in Oceanside, California. Drink one cup every 3 hours.

Ginger can help reduce pain and inflammation. Licorice provides a pleasant taste and is thought to aid the immune system against viruses. Echinacea boosts the body's immune system. Goldenseal is used to fight bacteria. Honey is a sweet-tasting antibacterial and antimicrobial.

1 piece fresh ginger (5" long by ½"–1½" thick), finely chopped
1 tablespoon dried licorice root
6 cups water
20 drops echinacea tincture
20 drops goldenseal tincture
1 tablespoon honey

Combine the ginger, licorice root, and water in a saucepan. Bring to a boil. Cover and simmer on low heat for 20 minutes. Strain and add the echinacea and goldenseal tinctures and honey.

Sip marshmallow tea. To soothe and moisten a dry, irritated throat during the day, sip on marshmallow root tea. To make the tea, put ¼ cup of dried, chopped marshmallow root in a glass or ceramic jar. Then pour 1 pint of room-temperature water over it. Cover the jar and allow the herb to steep overnight. In the morning, strain, and add 4 teaspoons of honey to the liquid. Sip ¼ to ½ cup of tea at a time throughout the day. The mixture is good for only 1 day, so drink as much as you can in a day and dispose of the rest.

Stress

Sometimes, the smallest thing can unleash feelings of tension and stress: the alarm clock that didn't go off. A cup of coffee spilling into your lap. Bumper-to-bumper traffic. Work deadlines. Family demands. The dog that overturns the trash can. The list is endless.

Simply put, stress is any pressure that disrupts the regular rhythms of your life and emotions. This pressure can come in the form of a physical complaint, such as a cold or an aching knee joint. It can be purely emotional, like worry over a pressing deadline or anger about a romantic breakup. Or it can be an assault from without, such as a noisy party next door or a frightening thunderstorm.

Any of these stresses can leave you feeling depressed, irritable, edgy, or anxious. Sustained stress can elevate your blood pressure, weaken your immune system, trigger headaches and backaches, and raise your risk for a host of serious disorders, such as heart disease.

Knowing healthy ways to unshackle stress's grip gives you more control over life's expected—and unexpected—challenges. Relaxation techniques, deep breathing, physical activity, getting enough sleep, and eating well all can help you resist its ravages. Herbs can play a vital role, too. Botanical remedies won't make stress magically disappear, but they can be a helpful addition to your personal stress-management plan.

Create serenity with an herbal formula. If you face a seriously stressful situation, you can ease your body and your mind quickly with this blend. Combine two parts each of tinctures of skullcap and valerian with one part each of tinctures of chamomile, mugwort, and motherwort. Take a teaspoon of this blend as needed. Skullcap and valerian are traditional stress-relief herbs. Chamomile aids in digestion to prevent stomach upsets, mugwort is a gentle sedative, and motherwort helps you to relax and calms heart palpitations.

Unwind with a lavender bath. If you've had an especially brutal, stressful day, help ensure a good night's sleep by first soaking in a lavender bath. Essential oils aren't soluble in bathwater, but they do dissolve in milk, so add 1 to 5 drops of lavender essential oil to ½ cup of milk. Pour this mix into a tub of comfortably warm water and relax. Make sure you select the *Lavandula angustifolia* species of this herb, which is noted for its floral, relaxing scent.

Bust stress with aromatherapy. To elevate your mood when stress strikes, tailor the aroma of essential oils to your personal needs. Concoct a take-along bottle of stress-busting smelling salts by combining 1 tablespoon of coarse rock salt with 6 drops of essential oil in a bowl. Mix well. Transfer to a small, dark glass bottle with a tight-fitting lid. When you feel stressed, open the bottle and gently fan the fragrance with your hand toward your nose. Then sit back, close your eyes, and breathe deeply.

Which essential oils should you choose? For tension, try lavender and orange; for anger and irritability, use bergamot and chamomile; for anxiety, try cedar and ylang-ylang.

Stress-proof with Siberian ginseng. To protect your body from the effects of stress, herbalists recommend taking ½ to ¾ teaspoon of Siberian ginseng tincture three times per day. Take the herb daily for 6 weeks, followed by a 2-week break, then resume for as long as necessary. Siberian ginseng contains at least 18 different hormone-like saponins, which botanists say fight stress and fatigue.

Stretch Marks

Although stretch marks are most often associated with pregnancy and weight gain, other factors can stretch the skin's elastic tissue to the max, leaving behind those unmistakable lines.

Exercises that bulk up muscle can do it. So can prolonged use of high-potency cortisone creams and other corticosteroid medications.

Stretch marks initially appear as pinkish or purplish lines on the breasts, abdomen, buttocks, thighs, and sometimes the arms. Gradually, they lighten or turn white and shiny.

Once you have these scarlike marks, they stick around for a lifetime. Moisturizers, wrinkle creams, and massages won't make them vanish, say medical experts. But you can take steps to avoid getting more stretch marks, with good nutrition, regular exercise, and the following herbal remedy.

Rub on skin balm. Minimize or even avoid stretch marks before they happen by rubbing this herbal balm into skin that you know will be stretched. Combine 4 ounces of almond oil or a blend of almond and olive oil with a few drops of lavender essential oil and an ounce or more of calendula infused oil.

The best application method is to rub this herbal balm all over the area daily. The oils and herbs will help keep the skin supple and help it stretch without leaving stretch marks. Lavender essential oil is soothing and antimicrobial, while calendula contains skin-healing properties.

Sunburn

Whether you're on the golf course, at the beach, or working in your garden, the sun's ultraviolet rays initially feel invitingly warm on your skin. But overexposure to the sun can leave unprotected skin painfully tender, red, swollen, and even blistery.

What's going on? Medical experts say that the blood vessels near your skin's surface dilate in response to too much sun. Anyone can get a sunburn, but fair-skinned people and

Spray Away Sunburn Pain

Both lavender essential oil and the gel of the aloe vera plant can reduce inflammation and soothe tender, sunburned skin. Combine the healing and cooling powers of both in this sunburn spray created by Mindy Green, a founding and professional member of the American Herbalists Guild and director of educational services for the Herb Research Foundation in Boulder, Colorado.

In a small spritzer bottle, mix together 50 drops (about ½ teaspoon) of lavender essential oil, 4 ounces of aloe vera juice, 1 teaspoon of vitamin E oil, and 1 tablespoon of vinegar. (Lavender essential oil, aloe vera juice, and vitamin E oil are all available at health food stores.)

Shake well before each use. Spray as often as needed to reduce sunburn pain. Store the bottle in the refrigerator to chill the spray and enhance the cooling sensation on your skin.

those with blond, red, or light brown hair are at the greatest risk for sun-related skin damage. Some medications and some herbs can increase sun sensitivity, too.

Minimize sunburns by heeding these rules. Avoid direct sunlight from 10:00 A.M. to 3:00 P.M., when the sun's harmful rays are the strongest. And stay covered with a brimmed hat, longer shorts, long-sleeved shirts, and sunglasses. Apply sunblock with a sun protection factor (SPF) of 15 or higher.

If your sunburn is so severe that you have blisters, a fever, chills, or severe pain, you could have sun poisoning. Get medical attention immediately. These symptoms can also indicate the possibility of heat exhaustion or heatstroke.

For routine sunburn, try these herbal offerings to relieve the pain, reduce the swelling, and hasten the healing.

Make aloe your ally. For immediate treatment of minor sunburn, herbalists suggest you cut or snap off a leaf from a mature aloe plant. Cut it down its length and squeeze out the transparent gel from inside the leaf directly onto your sunburned skin. Aloe forms a coating on the surface of your skin that helps prevent dehydration from the inside out, which can help reduce blistering. This healing gel also contains vitamins C and E as well as zinc, all of which are nutrients that speed burn healing. Research demonstrates that fresh aloe gel reduces inflammation and appears to enhance skin repair when applied to burns.

Pat yourself with black tea. To subdue sunburn pain as soon as it starts, rely on the tannic acid in tea. Make a cup of regular black or orange pekoe tea and let it cool. Then pat it on your sunburned skin. You can use your fingertips or soak a cotton ball in the tea and apply. The tea's tannic acid helps restore the natural acid balance of your skin, which helps protect against infection. These tannins also activate proteins in the top layers of your skin to form a protective covering and help dispel the feeling of heat. Reapply this tea as needed.

Soak in apple-cider vinegar. If your sunburn covers your body, fight the heat and pain by bathing in apple-cider vinegar. To prepare the bath, add a cup of apple-cider vinegar to a tubful of cool water. Relax, soak, and allow the astringent properties of the apple-cider vinegar to ease your pain.

Toothaches

Toothaches are like the class bully back in grammar school: impossible to ignore. You can try bypassing a painful tooth by chewing with the other teeth, but one false chew and—*ouch!*—the injured tooth delivers a jolt of pain.

Teeth ache because bacteria-laden plaque invades beneath the gum line, eventually irritating oh-so-sensitive nerve endings. Beyond pain, this plaque assault can leave behind cavities, tooth decay, or an abscess. So heed the pain warnings and see your dentist pronto. In the meantime, try one of these herbal pain relievers to help you through the rough spots.

Stop pain with a dab of clove. To temporarily quell throbbing tooth pain, rub a drop of oil of clove directly on the aching tooth. If you don't have this oil handy, reach for a whole clove from your spice rack and rub the pointed end on the teeth closest to the aching area. Oil of clove contains 60 to 90 percent eugenol, a potent pain-deadening antimicrobial. Clove has earned the official endorsement of the Food and Drug Administration as an effective stopgap measure for tooth pain.

Compress pain with ginger. Diminish deep toothache pain by making a compress with ginger. This hot spice acts as a counterirritant, effectively distracting you from toothache pain. To make a compress for your aching tooth, mix a little powdered ginger in enough water to create a gooey paste. Dip a small cotton ball in the paste, then apply it directly to the tooth, trying not to get the paste on the gum. If you don't have ginger available, use cayenne pepper, following the same instructions. Cayenne contains salicylates, aspirin-like pain-subsiding chemicals.

Rely on this Chinese folk remedy. Since the fourth century, the Chinese have been reaching for sesame seeds to subdue tooth pain. Herbalists say sesame contains at least seven pain-relieving compounds. For best results, boil one part sesame seed with two parts water until half the liquid remains. Cool the resulting decoction and apply it directly to your aching tooth.

Munch willow bark. For short-term relief from toothaches, chew on a small wad of willow bark. Willow bark contains salicin, a chemical cousin of aspirin that shares its pain-relieving powers. You can also drink a tea

---

THE HERBAL KITCHEN

Peppermint Toothpaste

When she was a child, herbalist Rosemary Gladstar made regular trips to the dentist to have cavities treated. By the time she reached early adulthood, she needed root canal work. Fortunately, she found a way to bring her dental problems under control.

"About 15 years ago, I started making my own herbal toothpaste, and it has really cut down on my dental problems. Its alkalizing effect seems to reduce infections in my mouth," says Gladstar, who is director of the Sage Mountain Herbal Education Center in East Barre, Vermont.

Gladstar's herbal toothpaste keeps well, so store it in a closed glass container on your bathroom sink. The peppermint provides mouth-freshening flavor, while the goldenseal and myrrh fight infection and receding gums.

- ¼ cup fine facial clay (available in health food stores)
- ¼ cup baking soda
- 1 teaspoon salt
- 1 teaspoon myrrh fine powder
- ¼ teaspoon goldenseal (organically cultivated powder form)
- 1–2 drops peppermint essential oil

Stir the clay, baking soda, salt, myrrh, goldenseal, and peppermint together in a bowl. Add water, a few drops at a time, until the mixture forms a paste. Apply a dab of the paste, then brush as usual. Rinse.

made from this herb or take a tincture, following the label directions, to banish the ache.

Ulcers

Medical experts used to blame ulcers on stress, smoking, drinking excess alcohol, and eating rich or spicy foods. While any of these factors can cause pain, the scientific community has now found another, more common cause of ulcers themselves: a spiral-shaped bacterium answering to the name of *Helicobacter pylori*.

These airborne bacteria are still something of a mystery. Researchers aren't certain where they come from or how infection occurs. But scientists do know that they settle in the stomach or top part of the small intestine, where they penetrate the digestive tract's protective lining.

Whether your ulcer is the result of a bacterial invasion, stress, or lifestyle habits, the consequences are the same. Acid eats away at your stomach or intestinal lining, leaving a painful sore. People with ulcers often experience a gnawing or burning pain in the abdomen, usually between meals or first thing in the morning. Some also vomit, lose weight, lose their appetite, develop blood in their stools, and feel nauseated.

It's important to see your doctor first for ulcer treatment. You can be tested for the presence of *Helicobacter pylori* and given medication to get rid of it. If that isn't the cause, or if you want to give your body extra help in getting over a bout of painful ulcers, herbalists recommend these remedies, which hasten healing and lessen the likelihood of repeat episodes.

Chew some licorice. To reduce the chances of recurring ulcers, take a natural product called deglycyrrhizinated licorice (DGL). Before or between meals slowly chew two tablets of DGL extract or swallow ½ teaspoon of the powder form. Stay on this herbal remedy for as long as symptoms persist. This herb contains several anti-ulcer compounds that protect the lining of the stomach and small intestine.

Sip anti-ulcer tea. Turn the volume down on ulcer pain, natural healers say, by drinking up to 2 cups of this herbal tea every day until your condition improves. Blend 1 teaspoon each of the dried herbs licorice root, marshmallow root, and chamomile flowers with ½ teaspoon each of Oregon grape root, hops, echinacea, and cinnamon in a pan with 1 quart of water. Bring to a boil, then simmer for 15 minutes. Remove from the heat and steep for 10 minutes. Strain the herbs and store the tea in the refrigerator until you're ready to drink it.

These herbs work in tandem to lower stomach acid levels, and they decrease the chances of a repeat ulcer attack.

Enjoy a fruit-and-spice drink. You can soothe a sore stomach by sipping a fruity anti-ulcer beverage between meals. Put blueberries and a banana in a blender. Add ground cinnamon, ground cloves, and ground ginger to taste. Blend until smooth and garnish each serving with a peppermint sprig. The tasty, no-fat ingredients in this recipe all contain significant amounts of stomach-soothing, ulcer-fighting compounds.

Urinary Tract Infections

When you gotta go, you gotta go. But if you have a frequent, urgent need to urinate accompanied by a burning sensation or pain in your urethra—the little pipe through which your urine exits—you may have a urinary tract infection (UTI).

Urinary tract infections occur when bacteria invade

> **• Herb at a Glance •**
> **Slippery elm.** Good for irritation and inflammation of the reproductive, digestive, and respiratory systems as well as of the urinary tract

the urethra. Less-than-sanitary toilet habits contribute to getting UTIs. So does using diaphragms and spermicides as well as douches or feminine deodorants. For women, peak times for these infections generally are just before menstruation, following intercourse, and at menopause, when the vaginal walls are more susceptible to bacteria.

Although men get UTIs, women are eight times more likely to suffer them. And one bout of infection increases the odds for more. You can lower your chances of a future UTI attack by practicing good hygiene, such as wiping from front to back after you use the toilet. This keeps bacteria away from the urethra. Drink up to eight glasses of water per day and urinate as needed. Holding back only allows bacteria to grow.

Visit your doctor if you see blood in your urine, which is an indication that you may have a more serious bladder or kidney condition. Most likely, your doctor will give you antibiotics to kill the bacterial invaders that caused the infection.

If you're otherwise healthy, UTIs usually clear themselves within 3 to 7 days. But most people don't want to endure the pain that long. Turn to these herbal helpers, which outwit the bacteria and fortify the mucous membranes that line the urinary tract against infection. Since a prolonged urinary tract infection can damage your kidneys, it is important to see a doctor if a UTI doesn't clear after 7 days.

Drink plenty of cranberry juice. To prevent bacteria from sticking to bladder walls, herbalists suggest drinking up to 17 ounces of cranberry juice per day. Scientific studies show that this fruit contains arbutin, a chemical compound that acts as both an antibiotic and a diuretic.

Try an antiseptic formula. Fight infection and soothe urination pain with uva-ursi, corn silk, and echinacea. Herbalists recommend taking 10 drops of each herb in tincture form in ½ cup of water or a noncitrus juice as needed. Drink this natural antiseptic to kill bacteria in your urinary tract. Don't use uva-ursi for more than 2 weeks without the supervision of a qualified herbalist. Also, don't use it if you have kidney disease because it contains tannins, which can cause further kidney damage. Tannins can also irritate your stomach.

Bathe in relief. To relieve the external burning of a UTI and hasten healing, sit in a tub that's half-filled with warm water and a few drops of essential oils, natural healers recommend. In a small dish, combine 3 drops of sandalwood essential oil, 2 drops of tea tree essential oil, 1 drop of chamomile essential oil, and 2 tablespoons of honey. Pour 2 tablespoons of apple-cider vinegar, which is a mild astringent, into the bath and then add the honey mixture, which helps hold the oils together and keeps them from floating on top of the water. Soak for 20 minutes.

Sandalwood is antibacterial, tea tree is antiseptic, and chamomile is anti-inflammatory.

Vaginal Dryness

Sex should feel wonderful. But intercourse can be downright painful if your vagina isn't well-lubricated, a condition that may be temporary—if you're breastfeeding, for example—or, if the result of natural hormonal changes, long-lasting.

After menopause, the vaginal lining thins and dries because of dwindling supplies of the female hormone estrogen. Estrogen helps keep vaginal tissue moist and healthy. In addition, menopause causes the vagina to shrink and lose muscle tone.

While vaginal dryness poses no serious health threat, it does make sex uncomfortable—and, sometimes, impossible. Here are some herbal solutions to help keep your love life flowing.

Try this aloe-powered liquid lube. Keep your vagina well-lubricated with this herbal "moisturizer," suggest natural healers. Blend equal parts of distilled witch hazel and pure aloe vera gel. For added slickness, mix in some slippery elm powder, say herbalists. Use as needed before and during sex.

Apply rejuvenation oil. Moisturize your vagina with an herbalist-recommended vaginal rejuvenation oil blend. Combine 2 ounces of almond oil or vegetable oil, 6 drops each of rose geranium and lavender essential oils, and 1,500 international units (IU) of vitamin E oil. (You can use the oil from vitamin E capsules.) Apply this oil blend inside the vagina as needed to restore moisture. *Note:* Don't use oil with latex forms of birth control, such as condoms.

Vaginal Itch

Few things are as maddening as vaginal itching, which is equally uncomfortable and embarrassing.

Itching may be a sign that you have a yeast infection, a bacterial infection, or even a sexually transmitted disease such as chlamydia, herpes, or gonorrhea. Or the delicate skin in and around your vagina may be reacting to chemicals in douches, bubble baths, or soaps. Changes in hormone levels, especially before menstruation, during pregnancy, while breastfeeding, and after menopause, can also cause that itchy feeling.

Medical experts advise against treating a vaginal itch on your own unless you know exactly what you're dealing with. Check with a doctor to pinpoint the cause. Often, he will prescribe antibiotics or a vaginal cream to prevent complications and soothe the irritation quickly. After you've seen your doctor and have your medical prescriptions, try these botanically based helpers to assist in relieving itching and discomfort.

Stop the itch with Caladium. Reach for relief with homeopathic Caladium, a remedy herbalists highly recommend. Take a 6X dose up to three times a day for no longer than 3 days. But if it is not helping after three doses, discontinue use because it's probably not the right remedy for your condition. The notation 6X is a standard measurement in homeopathy and refers to a remedy's potency, which is listed on the label.

Soak in apple-cider vinegar. To banish many types of vaginitis, add 3 cups of apple-cider vinegar to a hot bath. Soak in the tub for at least 20 minutes, spreading your legs to allow the water to flow around your vagina. Herbalists say vinegar baths help restore normal vaginal acidity.

Varicose Veins

The veins in your legs are among the longest in your body. When they're working properly, a series of 10 to 20 tiny valves inside them act like locks in a canal, allowing blood returning to the heart to collect at various points and then move on its way.

But sometimes, good veins go bad. Valves weaken, allowing blood that was headed up to your heart to trickle back down and pool instead. As a result, sections of your veins swell.

The word *varicose* means "swollen." Because they're extremely dilated, varicose veins seem to nearly pop from the skin. They're most noticeable in the legs since standing upright exerts tremendous pressure on the blood vessels down there. Women are four times more prone to varicose veins

> • *Herb at a Glance* •
> **Spearmint.** Good for indigestion during pregnancy and combating midafternoon slumps

than men are, perhaps because pregnancy increases pressure on the veins in the legs. Obesity, aging, and standing for hours on the job also cause vein swelling.

In most instances, varicose veins can make your legs feel tired, tight, and heavy. In rare cases, this condition can lead to a blood clot. If you experience sudden, painful swelling of one leg with tenderness in the calf muscle, seek medical help right away. A blood clot may have formed in one of the deep veins of your leg.

If you have garden-variety varicose veins or if you want to avoid developing them in the first place, these herbs can help keep your blood vessels strong and elastic, improve circulation, and make those purple bulges less unsightly.

Choose bilberry for stronger veins. If you want to improve the appearance of varicosity and strengthen your leg veins, take 80 milligrams of bilberry in capsule form three times a day—at breakfast, lunch, and dinner. Bilberry restores the connective tissue sheath surrounding veins. This prevents the veins from bulging, so excess blood won't start to collect. In addition, bilberry helps circulation by stimulating new capillary formation and strengthening capillary walls.

Ease the bulge with an herbal formula. Prevent existing varicose veins from getting any worse with this herbalist-recommended recipe. Combine two parts ginkgo tincture, one part ginger tincture, and one part cinnamon tincture. Take 30 drops of this combination, mixed with a liquid (such as tea, juice, or water), three times per day.

After a month, reevaluate your condition. You may or may not need to use the formula a little longer. Cinnamon is an herb that increases circulation. Ginkgo is a highly regarded treatment for a variety of blood vessel disorders. Ginger aids the cardiovascular system. It may make your gallbladder secrete more bile, however, so if you have gallstones, don't use therapeutic amounts of dried gingerroot or powder without guidance from a health care practitioner.

Go with a premade vein toner. A compound in horse chestnut helps to strengthen the capillary cells and reduce fluid leakage. Strengthening capillary tone can improve the appearance of varicose veins.

Horse chestnut is best used as a minor ingredient in an overall formula that includes other herbs. Look for commercial formulas of liquid tinctures or capsules that contain some horse chestnut—often, they are available by mail order.

Vomiting

Yes, it's unpleasant. But vomiting is often the most effective way for your body to eject harmful substances— from tainted food to too much alcohol. More often than not, you're better off letting it all out than suppressing a retch.

Fortunately, one good upchuck is usually all it takes to relieve nausea. But afterward, you may feel dehydrated, drained, and achy. Or you may be plagued by the dreaded dry heaves. That's when the herbal remedies listed below can help most.

If your vomiting goes on and on, however, check with your doctor to make sure you don't have a serious condition like toxicity, an infection of the digestive tract, or parasites.

Find relief in the spice rack. If the flu or tainted food causes repeat-performance vomiting as well as diarrhea, sip a tea made of cinnamon and ginger, herbalists suggest. Mix 1 teaspoon of dried cinnamon with ½ teaspoon of grated fresh ginger and add them to a cup of boiling water. Steep for 10 to 15 minutes, then strain and sip. Cinnamon is a natural astringent that dries up loose stools. Herbalists regard ginger as the premier herb for vomiting and nausea.

Calm with peppermint. A cup of peppermint tea can curb the muscle spasms in the digestive tract that often accompany vomiting. Mix a tablespoon of fresh peppermint leaves or a teaspoon of dried ones with a cup of hot water. Cover for 5 minutes to keep the healing volatile oils from escaping. Then strain and drink.

Soak up relief with an herbal bath. If nausea leads to vomiting, you might throw up any remedies you've swallowed. If that's the case, then try a soothing herb soak instead. Mix 1 tablespoon of fresh ginger or 1 teaspoon to 1 tablespoon of powdered ginger with a quart of just-boiled water. Let the water cool so you don't scald yourself, then soak your hands or feet until the vomiting subsides.

Warts

Usually painless, warts are nevertheless far from flattering. These knobby little skin lesions most commonly appear on the hands, fingers, forearms, knees, face, and feet.

Warts, which are actually benign skin tumors, are caused by a family of viruses called human papillomavirus (HPV). A suppressed immune system seems to increase susceptibility to warts.

Getting rid of warts doesn't always eliminate the virus that caused them in the first place, so natural healers suggest a two-pronged strategy for achieving a lasting solution: Bolster your immune system so that it can better battle viruses, and use herbs that work on the surface to shrink these little growths.

Wart Be Gone!

With just a drop or two a day of an easy-to-prepare recipe, you can make warts disappear.

The essential oils of tea tree and thuja possess antiviral and antifungal properties, making them powerful agents against warts, says Gail Ulrich, an herbalist, director of the Blazing Star Herbal School in Shelburne Falls, Massachusetts, and author of *Herbs to Boost Immunity*. Combined with a few other products, they make for a wonderful wart-dissolving oil.

You'll use only a little bit each day, so the solution should last for about 2 to 3 weeks. By then, the wart should be gone. You'll need castor oil, thuja essential oil, tea tree essential oil, and vitamin E capsules.

In a small wide-mouth bottle or jar with a lid, combine 1 tablespoon of castor oil, ¼ teaspoon of thuja essential oil, and ¼ teaspoon of tea tree essential oil. Using a needle, puncture two vitamin E capsules (each containing 400 international units). Squeeze out the vitamin E oil. Mix all the ingredients well.

Because the oil may burn the skin, cover the area surrounding the wart with a salve, such as vitamin E oil or lanolin. Using a cotton-tipped swab, a toothpick, or a dropper, apply the mixture to the wart. Place a bandage over the wart. Reapply the solution once a day until the wart disappears. Keep the solution in a covered bottle or jar, which you should store in a cool, dark place.

Bite back with birch bark. Make warts disappear safely and naturally with birch bark. People all over the world have relied on this herb for centuries. If you have access to fresh birch bark, tape a piece of moistened bark, with the inner side down, directly to the wart. If you can't get your hands on some bark, brew some birch bark tea by adding a teaspoon or two of powdered bark to a cup of boiling water. Steep for 10 minutes. You can drink it as a tea or rub it directly on the wart.

Birch bark contains two antiviral compounds, betulin and betulinic acid, in addition to salicylates, which are approved by the Food and Drug Administration to treat warts.

Fight the virus with echinacea. Fortify your immune system so that it can defeat wart viruses by taking two 250-milligram capsules of echinacea twice per day, natural healers recommend. Echinacea boosts immune system functioning.

Bombard with basil. Counter the HPV virus with crushed, fresh basil leaves. Simply pack the crushed leaves over the wart and cover with a bandage. Apply fresh basil daily for 5 to 7 days. This aromatic herb contains many antiviral compounds that have the potential to make warts disappear.

Water Retention

Swollen feet? Bloated abdomen? Fingers so puffy your rings get stuck? Most times, you can blame that bloated feeling on a lower level of the hormone progesterone. This decline usually occurs about a week to 10 days before your menstrual period begins.

As progesterone levels fall, your salt levels rise, so you retain water. The more salt you stock, the more water is retained throughout your body. Strange as it may sound, herbalists and conventional medical practitioners agree that you must actually drink *more* water to deflate water retention. At the same time, cut back on your salt intake. These front-line defenses help dilute sodium and assist your kidneys in flushing it out of your body.

Before trying herbal treatments, consult your doctor to find out exactly what's causing your water retention. Sometimes it's a symptom of a serious heart or kidney problem. If you have a condition called pitting edema, in which you've retained so much water that pressing on a swollen spot leaves an indentation on your skin, or if you retain water during pregnancy, it's also very important to contact your doctor.

If, on the other hand, you have a simple but irritating case of water retention, turn to the herbal pharmacy for gentle diuretics that help flush excess fluids from your body.

Diminish bloating with corn. If you're looking for a safe, effective diuretic, herbalists suggest corn silk tea. Steep 1 tablespoon of dried corn silk in a cup of just-boiled water for 5 minutes. Drink up to 3 cups per day, but avoid this herb at night—otherwise, you will be interrupting your sleep with trips to the bathroom.

Corn silk, the fine, threadlike strands jutting from the top of an ear of corn, prompts the kidneys to flush out excess water. Researchers aren't certain which compounds account for this fluid-flushing quality, but they know it works. Instead of sipping this tea, you could also use several cups of it as the flavorful base for vegetable soup. Don't use silk from store-bought corn for this tea, unless you know that it has been organically grown without pesticides. Otherwise, purchase corn silk in a health food store or by mail order from companies that sell organic herbs.

Drain with dandelion. Encourage more frequent urination, which eliminates extra fluid, by quaffing dandelion leaf tea, herbal healers suggest. Add 1 cup

> • *Herb at a Glance* •
> **Yarrow.** Good as a poultice for bleeding and wound healing

of boiling water to 1 teaspoon of dried dandelion leaf. Let it steep for 5 minutes before straining. Drink up to 3 cups per day for a few days before your monthly period is to start. If you are on medication, check with your doctor to make sure your medication is not a diuretic (something that causes fluid loss), as are certain blood pressure medications. If so, avoid dandelion.

Try an herbal combo. For variety, natural healers suggest this diuretic tea, which taps the effectiveness of both dandelion and corn silk as well as other diuretic herbs. Combine the following dried herbs: 2 teaspoons of dandelion root and ½ teaspoon each of nettle leaf, oatstraw, fennel seed, and corn silk. Add the herbs to a pot of boiling water. Cover, turn off the heat, and steep for 20 minutes. Strain and drink 1 to 2 cups per day as needed.

Wound Healing

You nicked your hand while pruning the hedge, and weeks later, it still hasn't healed completely. The scrape you got from a bicycle spill on gravel refuses to disappear. So does that little incision on your arm where the doctor removed a suspicious-looking mole.

In ideal conditions, a cut, scrape, or surgical incision mends swiftly and neatly. No sign of infection. No long-lasting red mark. No need to wear bandages for weeks on end. But conditions are often not so ideal. Everything from dirt and microbes to poor circulation can slow the healing process. Diabetes and hardening of the arteries— medical conditions that cause poor circulation—can also prevent wounds from healing. Don't try to self-treat a wound that won't mend, particularly if you have one of these conditions. See a doctor.

Otherwise, for a minor, nonthreatening wound, botanical remedies might help. Before using one, wash the injured site thoroughly with mild soap and water. Then enhance healing with these tissue-mending herbs.

Draw out debris with astringent herbs. If infection or small pieces of dirt slow healing, herbalists recommend an herbal soak. For wounds that you can easily immerse in a basin or large bowl, make a strong tea using 1 quart of water and ½ cup of either wild geranium, dried oak bark, or dried witch hazel. Simmer the tea for about 30 minutes, then strain. Soak the wound in the comfortably hot tea for at least 15 minutes to draw out debris and infection.

If the wound can't be soaked easily, use the strong tea mixture to make a compress. Soak a clean cloth in the tea, but don't wring it out. Lay the wet cloth over the wound. Every few minutes, rinse the cloth in the tea and reapply.

These astringent herbs have been used traditionally to clean wounds and make torn skin pull together. Combined with warm water, these herbs act like vacuum cleaners, sucking out debris.

Hasten healing with calendula. Once the wound is clean and infection-free, speed healing and lessen scarring with a calendula compress, herbalists suggest. Pour a cup of boiling water over 1 teaspoon of dried calendula petals and steep for 10 minutes. Then soak a clean cloth in the liquid and apply the cloth to the wound. Or you can buy commercial skin creams that contain calendula from health food stores. German medicinal herb experts endorse this herb to hasten skin healing.

Rely on echinacea. To fend off inflammation in hard-to-heal wounds, herbalists recommend a compress made with echinacea. Mix one part echinacea tincture with three parts water and apply to the wound with a clean cloth. Leave this compress in place for 10 to 15 minutes. Reapply four times per day until the wound is clearly healing.

Wrinkles

Wrinkles are a small price to pay for smiling at the skies as you watch hawks soar. Or laughing at a good joke. Or snuggling up to a big, fluffy pillow as you sleep.

In fact, if you've lived at all, you probably have wrinkles. The crinkles and creases usually start to surface after age 30 as collagen and elastin (protein fibers that give skin support and elasticity) start to break down.

Unprotected sun exposure is the most frequent cause of wrinkles; more than 90 percent of premature aging is a direct result of the sun's ultraviolet rays. The sun wreaks havoc on the skin by breaking down collagen and elastin, causing your skin to lose tone. Smoking also ages your skin prematurely, by constricting blood vessels and impairing circulation to the skin.

It's difficult to avoid or erase wrinkles completely, but there are plenty of lifestyle and herbal options that can minimize them. Drink plenty of water (at least eight 8-ounce glasses per day), don't smoke, wear sunscreen daily, avoid tanning salons, exercise regularly, and include some healthy fats in your diet, such as olive or canola oil. These lifestyle adjustments will give a glow and supple feeling to your skin. So can the following herbal wrinkle warriors.

Tame deep wrinkles with a botanical face treatment.
For pronounced wrinkles, use a strong botanical remedy made with lemon and water. Herbal treatments can remove the upper layers of dead skin and, over time, can minimize wrinkles by encouraging the growth of new skin, say herbalists. Before you apply this treatment, clean your skin with a nonoily cleanser. Make sure your hands are clean, too.

Mix equal parts of lemon juice and distilled water. Use your fingers to pat the mixture on your face, being careful

An Apple a Day Takes Wrinkles Away

Want a 25-cent alternative to the $75 bottles of alpha hydroxy acid cream sold to smooth out wrinkles? Then go to the grocery store and buy an apple.

Alpha hydroxy acids, which peel away layers of dead skin and expose the new skin underneath for a smoother appearance, naturally occur in fruits such as apples. Try using a homemade apple face mask to improve the condition of your skin, suggests Jenny McFeely, a member of Britain's National Institute of Medical Herbalists and a professional member of the American Herbalists Guild, who is from Scottsdale, Arizona.

Before making an apple face mask, clean your skin with a nonoily cleanser. Then cut up an apple and place it in a blender. Puree the apple until it is moist and pulpy. Smear it all over your face and leave it there for 15 to 20 minutes.

Use this treatment three times a week to get the same results you would expect from that expensive lotion that comes in a fancy bottle.

not to get any in your eyes or on your lips. Your face should feel a little puckery, and it may sting slightly. Leave the treatment on for 5 minutes, then rinse with lukewarm water and apply a nonpetroleum moisturizer. If you use a peel three times a week, small wrinkles may diminish within 3 months.

Concoct a natural face-lift. Tighten wrinkles temporarily with an egg facial, which will keep skin smooth looking for up to 5 hours. If you have oily skin, use only the egg whites. For normal or dry skin, use one whole egg. Whip the egg with 1 teaspoon of dried or fresh lavender flowers and apply to your clean face. Leave on until the egg hardens. Lay a wet washcloth (use tepid water) on your face to soften the egg. Then glide the egg off with the washcloth. Finish with a toner and a nonpetroleum moisturizer. This remedy works great when used before you go out to a special event where you want to look especially nice.

Safe Use Guidelines
for Herbs

While herbs are generally safe and cause few, if any, side effects, researchers and specialists in natural medicine caution that you should use them responsibly. Foremost, if you are under a doctor's care for any health condition or are taking any medication, don't take any herb without your doctor knowing about it. Certain natural substances can change the way your body absorbs and processes certain medications. Also, if you are pregnant, do not use any natural remedy without the consent of your obstetrician or midwife. The same goes for nursing mothers and women trying to conceive.

Below are cautions and guidelines for the herbs mentioned in this book that can potentially cause adverse reactions in some people. Though such occurrences are rare, you should be aware of what they are and discontinue use of the herb if you experience an unusual reaction. Also, do not exceed the recommended dosages—more is *not* better.

By familiarizing yourself with this list, you can enjoy the world of natural healing and use this book with confidence.

Aloe: Do not use gel externally on any surgical incision, because it may delay wound healing.

Angelica: Use sparingly and only for short periods of time. Increases sun sensitivity and may cause skin rash, so avoid prolonged sun exposure.

Arnica: Do not use on broken skin.

Basil: Do not take large amounts (several cups a day) for extended periods.

Bearberry: Do not use for more than 2 weeks without the supervision of a qualified herbalist. Do not use if you have kidney disease because it contains tannins, which can cause further kidney damage. Tannins can also irritate the stomach.

Birch: Do not take if you need to avoid aspirin since its active ingredient, salicin, is related to aspirin.

Black cohosh: Do not use for more than 6 months.

Black haw: If you have a history of kidney stones, do not take without medical supervision because it contains oxalates, which can cause kidney stones.

Bladderwrack: May reduce absorption of iron, sodium, and potassium, so do not take for more than 6 weeks. Not recommended if you have hyperthyroidism. Can aggravate existing acne.

Bloodroot: May cause nausea and vomiting in doses higher than 5 to 10 drops of tincture twice a day. Safe when used in commercial dental products.

Cayenne (ground red pepper): May irritate the gastrointestinal tract if taken on an empty stomach. Don't use near eyes.

Chamomile: May trigger an allergic reaction in people allergic to closely related plants, such as ragweed, asters, and chrysanthemums.

Chasteberry: May counter the effectiveness of birth control pills.

Coleus forskohlii: May enhance the effects of medications for asthma or high blood pressure with negative results, so do not use unless under medical supervision.

Coltsfoot: Do not use for more than 1 week unless under supervised care of a doctor or qualified herbalist.

Comfrey: For external use only. Do not use on deep or infected wounds because it can promote surface healing too quickly and not allow healing of underlying tissue.

Dandelion root: If you have gallbladder disease, do not use dandelion preparations without medical approval.

Dong quai: Do not use while menstruating, spotting, or bleeding heavily since it can increase blood loss.

Echinacea: Do not use if you're allergic to closely related plants, such as ragweed, asters, and chrysanthemums. Do not use if you have tuberculosis or an autoimmune condition such as lupus or multiple sclerosis because echinacea stimulates the immune system.

Ephedra: Do not use without the supervision of a medical doctor.

Eucalyptus: Do not use if you have inflammatory disease of the bile ducts or the gastrointestinal tract or severe liver disease. May cause nausea, vomiting, and diarrhea in doses higher than 4 grams a day.

Fennel: Do not use medicinally for more than 6 weeks without supervision of a qualified herbalist.

Feverfew: If chewed, fresh leaves can cause mouth sores in some people.

Flax: Take with at least 8 ounces of water.

Garlic: Do not use supplements if you are on anticoagulants or about to undergo surgery because garlic thins the blood and may increase bleeding. Do not use if you're taking hypoglycemic drugs.

Gentian: May cause nausea and vomiting in large doses. Do not use if you have high blood pressure, ulcers, or gastrointestinal irritation and inflammation.

Ginger: Dried root or powder used in therapeutic amounts may increase bile secretions in people with gallstones. Fresh ginger is safe when used as a spice.

Ginkgo: Do not use if you are taking antidepressant MAO inhibitor drugs, aspirin or other nonsteroidal anti-inflammatory medications, or blood-thinning medications. In doses higher than 240 milligrams of concentrated extract, it can cause rash, diarrhea, and vomiting.

Ginseng: May cause irritability if taken with caffeine or other stimulants. Do not take if you have high blood pressure.

Goldenrod: Do not use if you have a chronic kidney disorder.

Goldenseal: Do not use if you have high blood pressure.

Hawthorn: If you have a cardiovascular condition, do not take hawthorn regularly for more than a few weeks without medical supervision. You may require lower doses of other medications, such as drugs for high blood pressure. If you have low blood pressure caused by heart valve problems, do not use without medical supervision.

Hops: Do not take if you are prone to depression.

Horse chestnut: Can interfere with the action of other drugs, especially blood thinners. Can irritate the gastrointestinal tract.

Horsetail: Do not use the tincture if you have heart or kidney problems. May cause a thiamin deficiency. Do not take more than 2 grams per day of powdered extract or take for prolonged periods.

Jamaican dogwood: Do not exceed the recommended dose, and use only as needed.

Kava kava: Do not take with alcohol or barbiturates. Do not take more than the dose recommended on package. Use caution when driving or when operating equipment since this herb causes drowsiness.

Licorice: Do not use if you have diabetes, high blood pressure, liver or kidney disorders, or low potassium levels.

Do not use daily for more than 4 to 6 weeks because overuse can lead to water retention, high blood pressure caused by potassium loss, or impaired heart and kidney function.

Marshmallow: May slow the absorption of medications taken at the same time.

Meadowsweet: Do not use if you need to avoid aspirin since its active ingredient is related to aspirin.

Myrrh: Can cause diarrhea and irritation of the kidneys. Do not use if you have uterine bleeding for any reason.

Nettle: If you have allergies, your symptoms may worsen, so take only once a day for the first few days.

Oak: Do not use externally on extensively damaged skin.

Oatstraw: Do not use if you have celiac disease (gluten intolerance) because it contains gluten, a grain protein.

Psyllium: Take 1 hour after other drugs. Take with at least 8 ounces of water.

Rosemary: May cause excessive menstrual bleeding.

Rue: Can irritate the gastrointestinal tract and should not be used by individuals with poor kidney function. Can cause sensitivity to the sun.

Sage: In therapeutic amounts, it can increase the sedative side effects of drugs. Do not use if you have hypoglycemia or are undergoing anticonvulsant therapy. Safe when used as a spice.

St. John's wort: Can cause sensitivity to the sun. Do not use with antidepressants without medical approval.

Sarsaparilla: May speed elimination of prescription medications, thereby requiring an increase in their dose in order to be effective.

Sassafras: Long-term use of sassafras tea is not recommended. Do not take more than the recommended dose.

Shepherd's purse: Do not use if you have a history of kidney stones.

Tea: Fermented black tea is not recommended for excessive or long-term use because it is a nervous system stimulant. People with irregular heartbeats should limit their intake of green tea to no more than 2 cups daily because the caffeine and other alkaloids can speed up heart rates. Its bitter taste stimulates gastric acid production, so it should be consumed only in limited amounts by people with stomach ulcers.

Turmeric: Do not use therapeutically if you have high stomach acid levels or ulcers, gallstones, or bile duct obstruction. Safe for use as a spice.

Valerian: Do not use with sleep-enhancing or mood-regulating medications because it may intensify their effects. May cause heart palpitations and nervousness in sensitive individuals. If such stimulant action occurs, discontinue use.

Wild cherry: For occasional use only. Don't exceed recommended dose.

Willow: Because of their similar active ingredients, follow the same cautions with willow as you would for aspirin.

Yellow dock: If you have a history of kidney stones, do not take without medical supervision since it contains oxalates and tannins, which may adversely affect this condition.

Safe Use Guidelines
for Essential Oils

Essential oils are inhaled or placed on the skin, but they should never be taken internally because they're so concentrated that they can be toxic. One exception is peppermint oil, which can be ingested in capsule form. If you have gallbladder or liver disease, however, you shouldn't do so without a doctor's consent. Peppermint oil may also lead to stomach upset in sensitive individuals.

Never apply essential oils neat (undiluted) unless otherwise indicated. Dilute them first in a neutral base, which can be an oil (such as almond), cream, or gel. Many essential oils may cause skin irritation or allergic reactions in people with sensitive skin.

Before applying any new oil to your skin, always do a patch test. Put a few drops of diluted oil on the back of your wrist. Wait for an hour or more. If irritation or redness occurs, bathe the area with cold water. In the future, prepare a dilution with half the amount of essential oil or avoid it altogether. As with herbs, do not use essential oils without first consulting your doctor if you are pregnant or nursing. Essential oils should be stored in dark bottles, away from light and heat, and out of the reach of children and pets.

Angelica: Do not use topically if you have diabetes. When using the root oil, avoid direct sunlight because uneven skin coloring can occur.

Basil: May irritate the skin if used in a high concentration.

Bergamot: Avoid direct sunlight after topical application because uneven skin coloring can occur (except with the bergapten-free type).

Cedarwood: Use in moderation (no more than 2 weeks at a time). May irritate the skin if used in a high concentration.

Clove: Use in moderation (no more than 2 weeks at a time). This oil is used undiluted as anesthesia in dentistry.

Eucalyptus: Use in moderation (no more than 2 weeks at a time). May irritate the skin if used in a high concentration. Do not apply externally to the face.

Garlic: May irritate the skin if used in a high concentration.

Juniper: Use in moderation (no more than 2 weeks at a time). Do not use if you have kidney disease.

Lavender: Can be used neat, but keep it away from your eyes.

Lemon: May irritate the skin if used in a high concentration. Avoid direct sunlight after topical application because uneven skin coloring can occur.

Lemongrass: For topical use only. Do not inhale.

Orange: Avoid direct sunlight after topical application because uneven skin coloring can occur.

Peppermint: May irritate the skin if used in a high concentration. Do not use on your face.

Rosemary: Do not use if you have hypertension. Because of its powerful action on the nervous system, do not use if you have epilepsy.

Sage: Spanish sage can be used in moderation (no more than 2 weeks at a time), but do not use it at all if you have hypertension or epilepsy. Do not use clary sage with alcohol; this sage can cause a narcotic effect and exaggerate drunkenness. Do not use common sage at all.

Sandalwood: Can be used neat as a perfume, but keep it away from your eyes.

Tea tree: May be applied neat to the skin.

Thuja: Use cautiously. Not recommended for general use in massage oils, baths, or aromatherapy. May irritate the skin if used in a high concentration.

Thyme: Do not use red thyme. White and common thyme may irritate the skin if used in a high concentration and should not be used if you have hypertension.

Ylang-ylang: Can be used neat as a perfume, but keep it away from your eyes. Use in moderation since its strong smell can cause nausea or headaches.

Index

Underscored page references indicate boxed text.